THE NEW
ALKALINE
Diet & Cookbook

To Beat
KIDNEY Disease

By the author of:
THE KIDNEY HEALTH GOURMET
Nina Kolbe RD CSR LD
Board Certified Renal Dietitian

Other books by this author

Avoid Dialysis, 10 Step Diet Plan for Healthier Kidneys

Kidney Heath Gourmet, Diet Guide & Cookbook

See order form in back of this book.

Contents

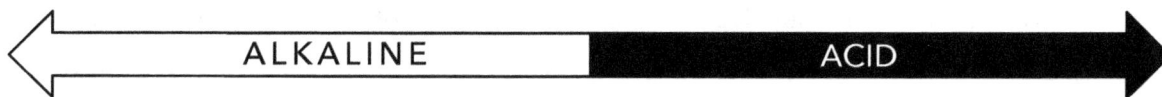

CHAPTER 1

Introduction

The renal diet for chronic kidney disease (CKD) has not changed significantly in recent years. The main nutritional-related goal for people with CKD has always been to slow the progression of kidney disease, minimize uremic toxins, and decrease protein in the urine. New research is promoting a new examination into how best we should manage diet in chronic kidney disease to reach this goal and minimize progression to end stage renal disease (ESRD). Toward that end, I have examined new research, many scholarly presentations, publications, focusing primarily on aspects of the CKD diet that could change the course of kidney disease. I am looking forward to sharing it with you. We are about to start a new treatment path that will result in the improved health of your kidneys.

Since I spend most of my days seeing patients in person, as I wrote this book, I wrote from the perspective that you the reader were sitting in front of me, chatting about the health of your kidneys.

Much of the scientific research behind the kidney diet has made marginal advances in the last several years. That is until now!!!. The lifestyle in this country has changed significantly. As I listen to patients in my office, I see the changes. Dining out used to be something one did to celebrate special occasions. Now eating out is a basic convenience and part of our social life. Restaurant or any convenience eating has also impacted our perception of what is a reasonable serving size. Our calorie, fat, sodium and chemical additives consumption have all dramatically increased. We consume food additives at alarming rates. These additives are found in convenience foods and processed foods.

Studies of changing meal patterns have identified that we eat snack foods possibly more than "real food". Unfortunately, as we eat more, we have decreased our physical activity. Modern con-

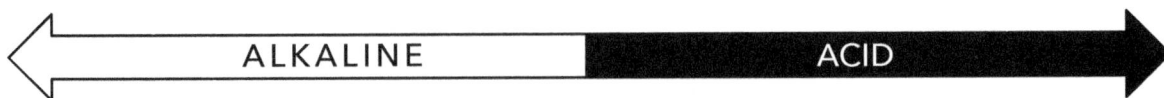

veniences are present in our daily lives. We take full advantage of robots vacuuming, car use for short trips, escalators or elevators for 1-2 flights of stairs. These changes have promoted the rapid rise of obesity. Statistically, 68.8% of the population is overweight and 35.7% obese, these changes contribute to many chronic conditions. 29 million people in the US have diabetes, half of the population in the US is either pre-diabetic or diabetic. If we look at the statistics for high blood pressure: 33% of the Caucasian population, 44% of African American population and 30% of Mexican American population is diagnosed with hypertension. Diabetes and high blood pressure are the two main contributors to the cause of chronic kidney disease.

Up to now, scientific literature has focused mostly on the American diet in terms of calories, sodium, fat, and sugar. Most recently scientists have drilled down to examine how the composition of our diet affects our organs, blood vessels and how making changes to meal patterns can decrease chronic diseases.

Exciting research has recently revealed how tweaking our meal choices can promote either an acidic or alkaline environment in our bodies. We have discovered how changes to our meal selection can put us in charge of our kidney health destiny.

The changes I will suggest may seem rather significant. Many readers will say "that's no problem, I can do that". Some may think it is too difficult to make the transition. Where ever you are in your meal pattern, any change you make will have positive health outcomes. Human behavior takes time to accept change, so it may be helpful to set small goals and celebrate your progress before setting the next small goal. I encourage you to take charge of your health destiny. Now to start, find yourself in the boxes below, can you make some dietary changes and move left. At a minimum, I would like for you to commit to following a Mediterranean diet as much as possible.

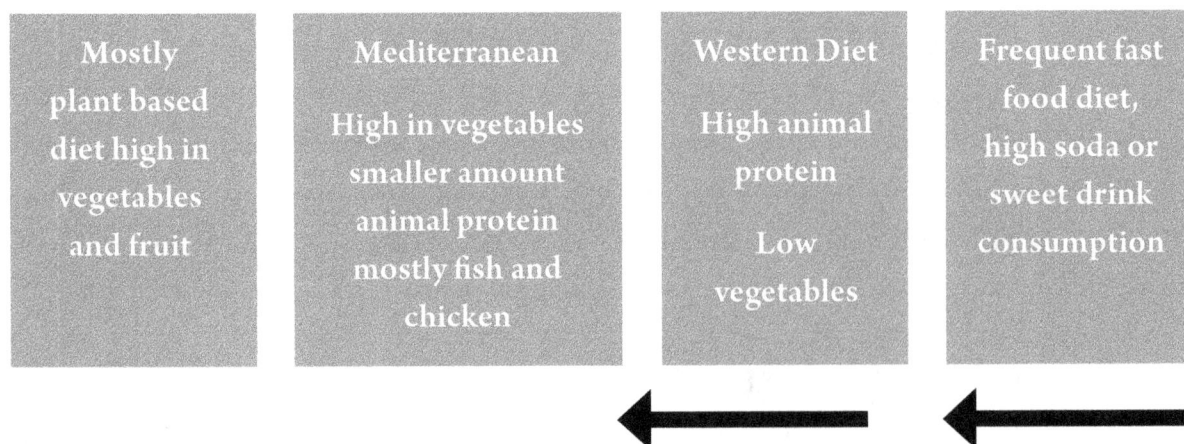

Mostly plant based diet high in vegetables and fruit	Mediterranean High in vegetables smaller amount animal protein mostly fish and chicken	Western Diet High animal protein Low vegetables	Frequent fast food diet, high soda or sweet drink consumption

◄   ◄

```
  ◀──────────── ALKALINE ───────── ACID ──────────▶
```

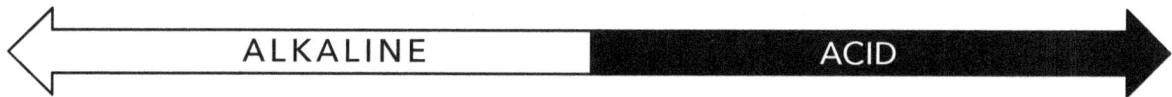

The Typical Western Diet

When we ask our family members what do you want for dinner? We are typically asking do you want beef, pork, chicken or fish. We plan our meals based on what we consider the main part of the meal, the center of the plate item. The starch portion comes second, and the vegetables are the tiny garnish on the plate, the afterthought.

This average western diet which is based on animal protein as the main component of the plate is setting in motion a cascade of events by promoting an acidic environment.

> **Animal protein promotes an acidic environment**
>
> **Vegetables promote an alkaline environment**

Animal protein is digested and broken down into acidic, sulfur-containing amino acids. Fruits and vegetables, on the other hand, are digested into an alkaline form which neutralizes acids in our kidneys.

A high animal protein diet promotes an acidic environment which in turn promotes a series of events setting in motion the stage for many chronic disease conditions.

Scientific studies have shown that a diet higher in dietary acid load is associated with a higher risk of protein found in the urine (albuminuria) an indicator of early kidney damage. Creating an alkaline environment has shown to benefit kidney health, blood pressure and other chronic disease conditions.

> **An alkaline environment in our blood benefits kidney health, blood pressure and other chronic diseases.**

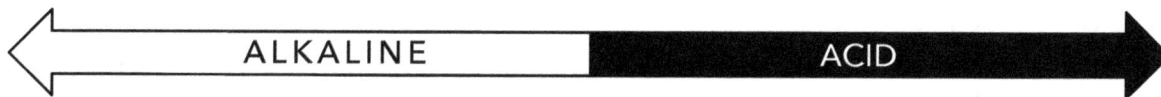

ALKALINE   ACID

CHAPTER 2

Acid-Base Simplified

What is pH?

Ph is a measure of the acidity or alkalinity of the body. While Ph balance is a balance between acid and alkali, both are important. The ideal pH of the body has a narrow range. A typical meat based western diet promotes a more acidic environment. *The term base is often interchangeable with alkali or alkaline all terms indicate that the food has a Ph of 7.35 or higher.*

How Our Diet Affects the pH

The Food Pathway; From the first bite to elimination:

Upon completion of a meal, the food particles are sent to the stomach for digestion and onto the small intestine for absorption of nutrients. The liquid waste will be eventually sent to the kidney for elimination. Each food item will be processed by the kidneys as either an acid forming substance or base forming substance. If we consume more acid promoting food than base forming food, we will contribute to an acidic environment.

> **A high animal protein diet creates an acidic environment**

```
←————————— ALKALINE ————————————— ACID —————————→
```

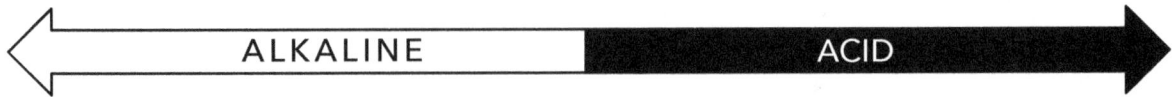

Acid-base and Your Kidneys

When we consume animal protein and digest it to its smaller component of amino acids, sulfur is released and urea is formed. Sulfur is acidic and in response to this acid environment the kidneys are prompted to increase ammonia production to buffer this acidic environment.

In an individual with decreased kidney function, a high dietary acid load promotes mechanisms to increase acid excretion. The kidney is working harder to manage the acid load while it has a reduced number of nephrons (basic functional unit of the kidney).

> The kidneys work harder to
> get rid of excess acid

Our western diet, high in animal protein, leads to increased ammonia production to buffer the acidic environment. Over time the excess ammonia is excreted via the kidneys. As we continue to consume sulfur containing, acidic amino acids, we rely on ammonia to buffer this acidic environment. This continued ammonia excretion leads to renal tubule-interstitial injury and metabolic acidosis.

Metabolic Acidosis

Is a common complication of moderate to severe CKD that results from impaired renal acid excretion. Several studies have shown that this metabolic acidosis is associated with a progression of kidney disease. Other studies have shown that treating this acidosis by increasing fruits and vegetables, slowed progression of CKD.

> Add balance to your meals
> Eat less acid promoting foods: meat, eggs and cheese
>
> Eat more base promoting foods: fruit and vegetables

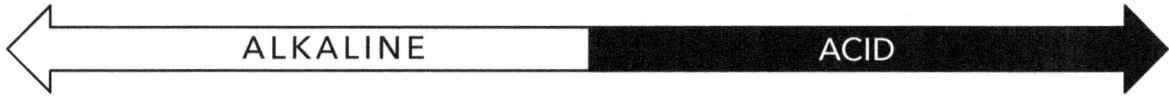

ALKALINE | ACID

CHAPTER 3

Prevent Metabolic Acidosis with Vegetables and Fruits

In a chronic kidney disease study, Dr. Donald E. Wessen and colleagues at Texas A&M College of Medicine, studied the effect of adding fruits and vegetables to the diet. The effect on different bio markers in CKD patients were tested. 71 study subjects with stage 4 CKD were selected to receive added fruits and vegetables for a period of 1 year. The focus was to compare the effects of alkali therapy by using fruits and vegetables or standard alkali therapy using bicarbonate, which has traditionally been used to treat CKD patients with metabolic acidosis. **The finding was that adding fruits and vegetables was as effective as bicarbonate in lessening metabolic acidosis.**

> The fruits and vegetable group did not have a rise in blood potassium level despite consuming more vegetables.

Dr. Wessen found that adding fruits and vegetables improved metabolic acidosis in stage 4 CKD. This, in turn, promoted better blood pressure control and lower urine sodium excretion. In addition, consuming more fruit and vegetables also caused the study participants to decrease their intake of processed foods; Which decreased sodium intake, promoting improved blood pressure control.

Adding more fruits and vegetables improved snack habits in the study participants. Fewer processed snacks led to better calcium and phosphorus levels in the study group.

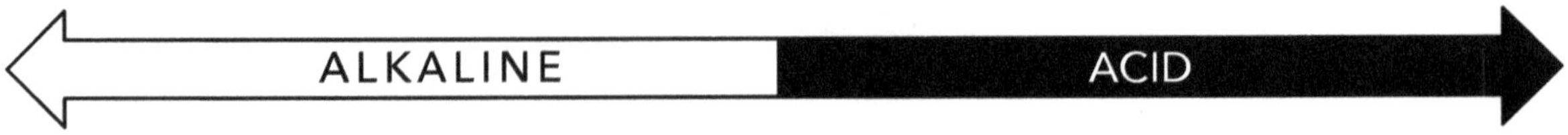

ALKALINE | ACID

This does not mean that you should stop eating all foods which promote an acidic environment, but the aim is for a more balanced plate.

In summary the benefit of adding vegetables and fruit to the diet:

- Decreases acidosis

- Improves blood pressure

- Improves calcium and phosphorus levels

- Improves snack habits

- Improves weight

- Adds vitamins, mineral and antioxidants

- Potential benefits to the immune system, cancer, eye health, bone health, heart disease, skin health and blood vessel health.

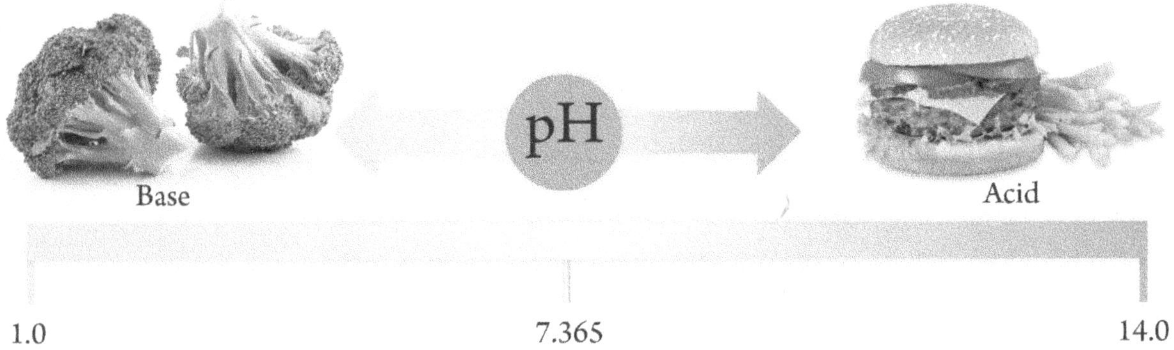

Base

pH →

Acid

1.0   7.365   14.0

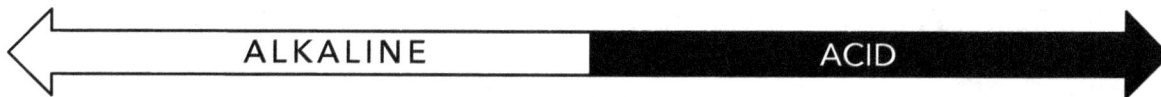

CHAPTER 4

Potential Renal Acid Load

We have Dr. Thomas Remer PhD and Dr. Friedrich Manz, MD to thank for developing a system which is called PRAL (potential renal acid load) and NAE (net acid excretion). Through a meticulous scientific process, a numerical number was assigned to a variety of foods. We can use these numbers to guide us in food selection.

The PRAL Score

The potential renal acid load of food (PRAL) is quantified in a number. If we used Dr. Remer's PRAL score to assess a typical American diet, it would indicate that we routinely select more foods which contribute to the acid load. This acidic state is not noticed on routine blood tests and medical visits. The negative impact is at the cellular level. To improve our health, we should set a goal of consuming more vegetable and fruit, alkaline promoting foods.

Use the PRAL score on the next several pages to plan meals which include more alkaline foods.

> To improve our health, we should set a
> goal of consuming more vegetables and fruit,
> alkaline promoting foods

Note how adding herbs and spices greatly improves the alkaline composition of your meal.

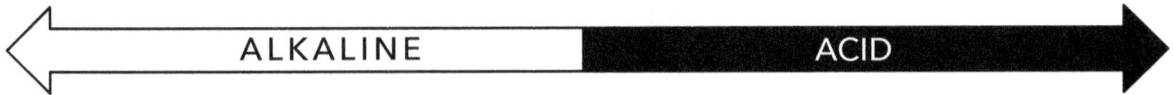

The Pral Score: Foods and dietary acid load: source USDA database.

Food	Very Alkaline	Quite Alkaline	Mostly Neutral	Quite Acid	Very Acid
Butter			.09		
Cheese (assorted)					16-21.0
Egg				9.41	
Egg substitute (whites)				2.50	
Milk		-1.02			
Milk-soy				.24	
Ricotta				5.80	
Yogurt				.11-.83	

CEREAL / PASTA				1.0-3.0	
Quinoa		-0.19			
Rice noodles				.97	
Rice (white and brown)				1.05	
Wild rice (cooked)				1.99	

COMMERCIAL BREAKFAST CEREALS				3-5.0	
Basic 4		-2.86			
Cheerios		-4.57			
Cooked Oatmeal				2.52-3.50	
Corn Chex		-2.84			
Familia		-3.74			
General Mills Raisin Bran	-27.58				
General Mills Total	-29.47				

ALKALINE ← | → ACID

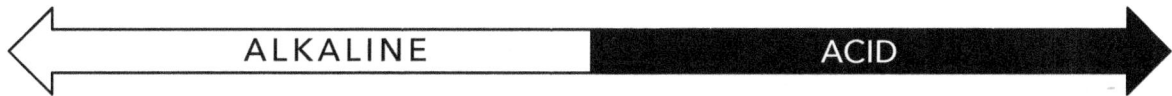

Food	Very Alkaline	Quite Alkaline	Mostly Neutral	Quite Acid	Very Acid
Kashi Go Lean				4.80	
Kashi Heart to Heart		-5.37			
Mixed grain oats				4.12	
Natures Path Optimum		-8.83			
Nature Valley Granola				6.55	
Peanut butter toast crunch		-3.48			
Smart Start Soy Protein		-0.52			
Wheaties				6.21	

POULTRY					
Fried chicken					11.22-14.0
Poultry, roasted					12.22-14.05
Turkey bacon					22.35

BEEF					
Ground beef					10.91-12.55
Liver					24.62
Ribs					17.93
Steak/roast					12.60-13.10

PORK					
Bacon, Canadian style					13.96
Bacon cured, baked					24.00
Bacon cured ,fried					26.00
Ham, cured					10.27-13.95

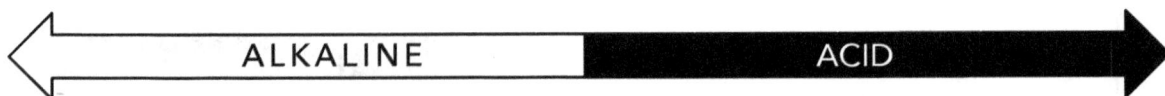

Food	Very Alkaline	Quite Alkaline	Mostly Neutral	Quite Acid	Very Acid
SEAFOOD					
Fish most varieties					9.0-10.0
Shrimp					10.10
Tuna canned in oil					20.45
Tuna canned in water					12.70
Tuna, cooked					18.14

Food	Very Alkaline	Quite Alkaline	Mostly Neutral	Quite Acid	Very Acid
Lunch meat					
Beef sausage				8.21	
Bologna				5.09-8.0	
Pastrami					11.59
Bratwurst sausage					10.27
Hot dog, beef				7.60	
Hot dog, chicken/turkey				7.03	
Ham, honey cured					19.24
Turkey breast meat				7.36	
Turkey ham					13.98
Turkey sausage					12.09

Food	Very Alkaline	Quite Alkaline	Mostly Neutral	Quite Acid	Very Acid
Vegetables					
Artichokes		-4.55			
Arugula		-4.97			
Asparagus		-1.44			
Bamboo shoots-		-9.12			
Kidney beans		-1.14			
Lima beans		-2.61			

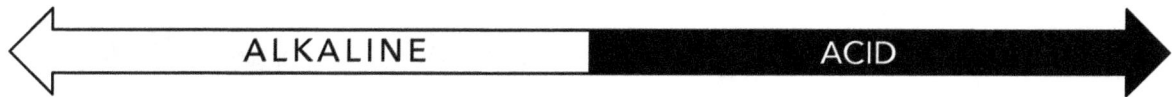

Food	Very Alkaline	Quite Alkaline	Mostly Neutral	Quite Acid	Very Acid
Navy Beans		-2.47			
Pinto Beans		-7.38			
Beans, green		-1.78			
Beet greens	-19.56				
Beets, canned solid		-2.67			
Black eyed peas		-0.80			
Broccolini		-5.17			
Broccoli		-3.28			
Brussel sprouts		-4.32			
Cabbage		-7.44			
Carrots		-4.30			
Cauliflower		-1.33			
Celery		-2.38			
Chard, Swiss		-8.14			
Chicory greens		-8.32			
Collards		-2.63			
Corn		-0.55			
Cucumber		-2.28			
Edamame		-1.50			
Eggplant		-1.98			
Endive		-6.01			
Fennel		-7.31			
Garlic		-2.64			
Ginger root		-7.89			
Kale		-4.22-6.15			
Kohlrabi		-5.41			

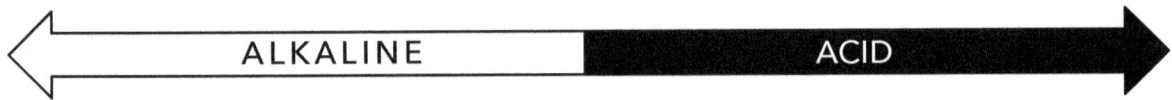

Food	Very Alkaline	Quite Alkaline	Mostly Neutral	Quite Acid	Very Acid
Lemongrass		-12.95			
Lentils				2.91	
Lettuce, Boston		-3.90			
Lettuce, romaine		-3.14			
Lettuce, iceberg		-2.19			
Mushrooms		-4.21			
Mushrooms, shitake dried	-20.21				
Mustard greens		-2.97			
Okra		-2.67			
Onions		-2.09			
Parsnip		-5.88			
Peas		-2.62			
Peppers, hot chili sun dried	-31.07				
Peppers, hot chili green		-3.31			
Peppers, jalapeno		-3.62			
Peppers, green		-2.75			
Peppers, red		-2.74			
Potato		-8.34			
Pumpkin	-10.90				
Radish		-4.40			
Rutabaga		-5.56			
Spinach	-10.28				
Squash, acorn		-8.65			
Squash, butternut		-3.51			
Squash, summer		-3.11			
Squash, zucchini		-4.26			

ALKALINE ← | → ACID

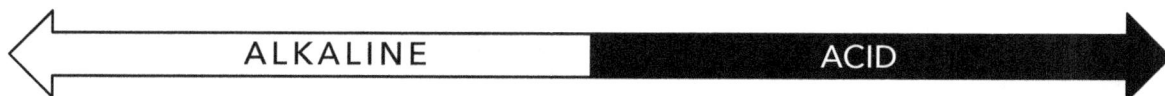

Food	Very Alkaline	Quite Alkaline	Mostly Neutral	Quite Acid	Very Acid
Sweet Potato		-2.51			
Tomato paste	-17.66				
Tomato, raw		-3.08			
Turnip greens		-1.14			
Yam	-15.11				
Yambean (jicama)		-2.21			

Fruit					
Apple		-1.92			
Apple juice		-2.38			
Apricots, dried		-7.90			
Apricots, fresh		-4.12			
Avocado		-8.19			
Banana		-6.93			
Blackberries		-2.90			
Blueberries		-1.49			
Clementine		-3.17			
Cranberries dried		-0.77			
Dates		-7.86			
Figs, dried		-6.06			
Grapefruit		-2.31			
Grapes		-3.64			
Kiwi		-6.12			
Lemon peel		-4.31			
Lime, raw		-1.71			
Mango		-2.98			

ALKALINE | ACID

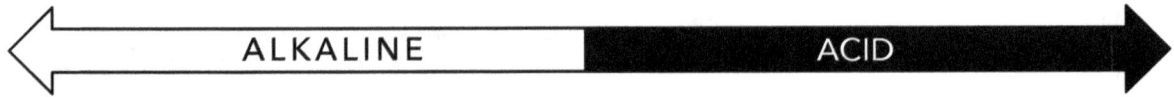

Food	Very Alkaline	Quite Alkaline	Mostly Neutral	Quite Acid	Very Acid
Melon, cantaloupe		-5.06			
Melon, honeydew		-4.45			
Nectarines		-3.05			
Olives, canned		-0.92			
Orange		-3.60			
Papaya		-5.48			
Peach		-3.11			
Pear		-2.14			
Pineapple		-2.33			
Plums		-2.62			
Raisins	-14.45				
Raspberries		-2.40			
Rhubarb		-3.72			
Strawberries		-2.54			
Tangerine		-3.14			

Fats and oils					
Butter, stick				0.63	
Margarine, spread			0.58		
Mayonnaise			0.06-		
Most Oils			0.0		

Herbs					
Basil, fresh	-10.01				
Capers, canned		-0.69			
Dill Weed, fresh	-15.49				

16

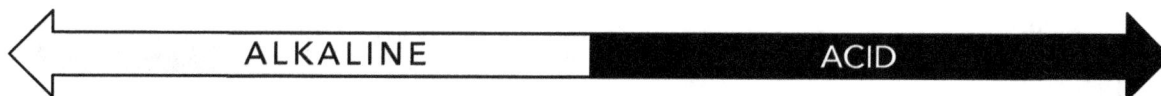

Food	Very Alkaline	Quite Alkaline	Mostly Neutral	Quite Acid	Very Acid
Horseradish		-4.87			
Mustard, yellow				1.13	
Peppermint, fresh	-12.65				
Rosemary, fresh	-16.45				
Table Salt		-0.50			
Spearmint, dried	-55.42				
Spearmint, fresh	-10.01				
Spice, allspice	-26				

Spices					
Anise	-18.17				
Basil, dried	-85.36				
Bay Leaf	-17.16				
Caraway Seed	-13.33				
Cardamom	-22.71				
Celery Seed	-34.40				
Chervil, dried	-92.40				
Celery, flakes	-84.46				
Chili Powder	-31.05				
Cinnamon	-23.75				
Cloves	-31.58				
Coriander	-99.48				
Cumin	-31.97				
Curry	-26.10				
Dill Seed	-33.19				
Dill Weed, dried	-74.51				

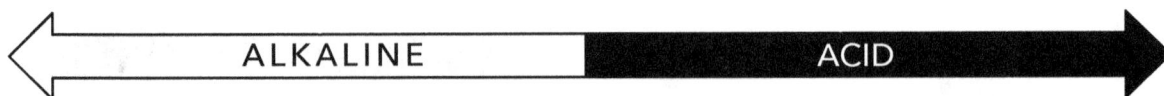

Food	Very Alkaline	Quite Alkaline	Mostly Neutral	Quite Acid	Very Acid
Fennel Seed	-35.37				
Fenugreek		-1.20			
Garlic, powder		-2.0			
Ginger, ground	-24.55				
Mace, ground	-9.87				
Marjoram, dried	-49.30				
Nutmeg		-3.75			
Onion, powder	-10.15				
Oregano, dried	-49.76				
Paprika	-36.33				
Parsley, dried	-81.49				
Pepper, black	-25.39				
Rosemary, dried	-37.43				
Saffron	-29.58				
Sage	-46.89				
Savory	-51.11				
Tarragon, dried	-64.51				
Thyme, dried	-46.66				
Thyme, fresh	-15.56				
Vinegar		-1.45			
Catsup		-6.67			
Nuts, assorted				2-6	
Seeds, flaxseed				2.13	
Sunflower Seeds					24.17

ALKALINE ——————————— **ACID**

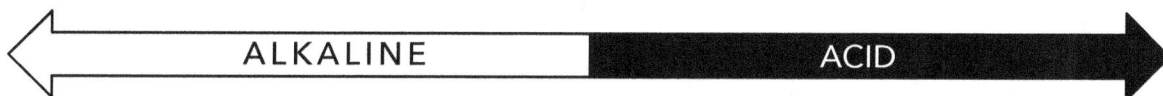

Food	Very Alkaline	Quite Alkaline	Mostly Neutral	Quite Acid	Very Acid
Beverages					
Beer			0.06		
Coffee		-1.20 - 4.0			
Distilled (vodka, rum, gin)				0.10	
Fruit drink powered with aspartame					16.65
Soda, Club		-0.13			
Soda, sweet				0.33	
Tea, brewed		-0.81			
Wine, red / white		-1.69 - 2.0			

Food	Very Alkaline	Quite Alkaline	Mostly Neutral	Quite Acid	Very Acid
Baked Goods					
Cakes, breads, cookies				4-6.0	

Food	Very Alkaline	Quite Alkaline	Mostly Neutral	Quite Acid	Very Acid
Fast Food					
Baked potato cheese and broccoli		-5.06			
Cheeseburger Hamburger				6.85 6.05	
Chicken Tenders / Chicken Sandwich					10.48
Eggs and Cheese Sandwich				6.38	
Fried fish				7.50	
Pizza				6.74	
Sub Sandwich with cold cuts				3.86	
Taco Salad				0.55	

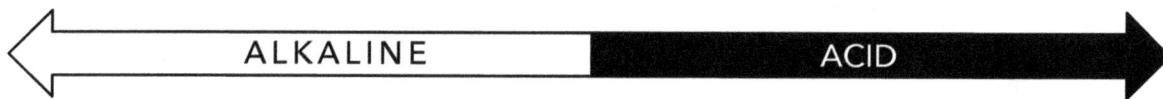

```
←  ALKALINE  |  ACID  →
```

CHAPTER 5

Alkaline Diet Improves Kidney Stones

Eating a plant based diet promoting an alkaline environment impacts the formation of kidney stones. The incidence of kidney stones has been rising dramatically with the increased consumption of animal protein, high fructose corn syrup sweetened beverages, obesity and sedentary lifestyle.

A standard diet prescription for "stone formers" is to reduce dietary intake of animal protein. Most kidney stones are composed of oxalate or calcium or a combination of both.

A study evaluated a vegetarian diet vs. standard diet on urinary oxalate and found decreased oxalic acid production in the study group following a vegetarian meal pattern.

> **An alkaline diet, plentiful in vegetables and fruits decreases oxalic acid and decreases the chance of forming kidney stones**

Sugar In the Diet Contributes to Kidney Stones

Another very popular part of the western diet, fructose, found in high fructose corn syrup used to sweeten beverages, also contributes to kidney stone formation.

ALKALINE   ACID

Drinking sodas and other beverages
sweetened with high fructose corn syrup
contributes to kidney stone formation

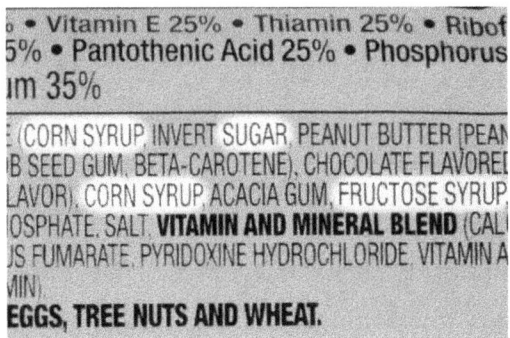

Increased fructose intake mostly from sweet beverages, which have a very high acid promoting PRAL score, increases the risk of forming kidney stones. High fructose corn syrup intake increases urinary oxalate, a risk factor for calcium oxalate kidney stones. Oxalate forms oxalic acid that also contributes to kidney toxicity.

I believe we are seeing a pattern, more animal protein and more fructose yields kidney producing toxins. More vegetables and fruits promote a soothing kidney friendly environment.

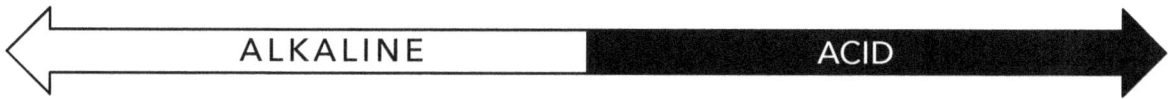

CHAPTER 6

Acidic Diet Gout and GUT

Uric Acid and Kidney Disease- the Chicken or the Egg.

High uric acid was commonly thought to be a consequence of chronic kidney disease. The decreased filtration of the kidney cells causing more uric acid accumulation. Researches are looking into whether it is actually the excessive uric acid which in turn is harming the kidneys.

> **Uric acid is formed from excessive animal protein intake and excessive sugar from high fructose corn syrup in beverages.**

The Link Between High Fructose Corn Syrup and Uric Acid

When we consume fructose in the form of high fructose corn syrup, the body breaks it down to chemical compounds called purines. Purine breakdown leads to the production of uric acid.

Studies have shown that within minutes of drinking a fructose corn syrup-sweetened soda, your uric acid levels rise.

As we consume fructose from sodas, candy, high fructose corn syrup beverages and other sweets, uric acid promotes fructose to be stored as fat and most often it is concentrated in the abdominal area, belly fat.

```
←————————— ALKALINE ————————|————————— ACID —————————→
```

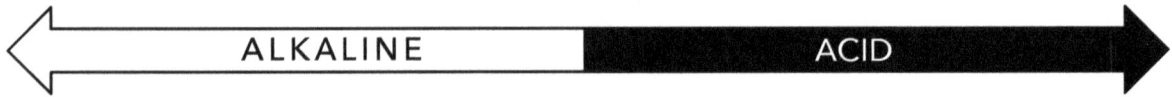

> **Within minutes of drinking a soda**
> **sweetened with high fructose corn syrup,**
> **uric levels rise**

How Is Uric Acid Harmful?

Consuming animal protein and high fructose corn syrup, lead to increased production of uric acid which can injure proximal renal tubules of the kidneys.

Uric acid can create a lot of mischief in the body. There is an association between high uric acid levels, high blood pressure, high blood sugar, abnormal cholesterol and or triglycerides and fat around the waist (metabolic syndrome) and stored fat in the liver (nonalcoholic fatty liver disease- NASH)

> **Fruits and vegetables lead to an alkaline**
> **environment decreasing uric acid.**
> **An alkaline diet helps the body break down**
> **uric acid and its excretion by the kidneys.**
>
> **Less uric acid, less toxicity to the kidneys!**

Uric acid is more soluble in an alkaline environment. The incidence of uric acid kidney stones and crystals are much higher in acidic urine.

Other factors which influence the amount of uric acid in the blood; Excess weight, lack of exercise and high animal protein, acidic diet.

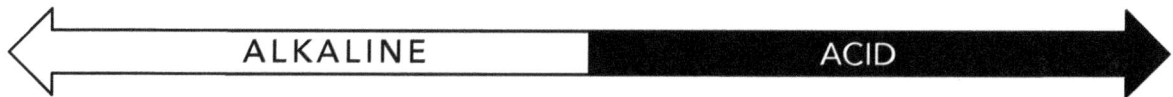

The GUT and the Kidney

The gastrointestinal track is found in the center of the body; it is home to over 100 trillion microbial cells. The gut serves an important role in processing nutrients we eat and disposing of waste. It also serves as a barrier to prevent entry of microbes and their harmful products into the internal environment of the body. Normal gut flora influences our health by maintaining balance of nutrition, metabolism, and immune function. Disturbing normal gut flora has been implicated with certain illnesses, such as obesity, type 2 diabetes, inflammatory bowel disease and cardiovascular disease. The toxins from "bad flora" have also been implicated as contributing to chronic kidney disease progression.

Eating more protein, creating an acidic environment feeds "bad bacteria" which thrive by feeding on uric acid and oxalates in the colon or large intestine.

> **Animal protein and high fructose corn syrup feed "bad bacteria"**

The effect of the uremic environment is worsened by inadequate intake of potassium containing fruits and vegetables.

> **Fruits and vegetables feed "good bacteria" and promote GUT balance**

Fruits and vegetables are the major sources of indigestible complex carbohydrates (fiber) that are the main source of nutrients for the normal gut bacteria, if potassium is limited the "good" bacteria lack nutrients and don't thrive, giving space to "bad uremic bacteria: profoundly affecting the gut microbiome. We now recognize the role of the altered gut microbiome in the progression and inflammation of chronic kidney disease.

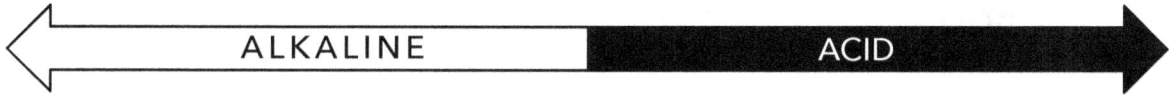

CHAPTER 7

All About Potassium

Potassium is an electrolyte that is vital to cell metabolism. It helps transport nutrients into cells and removes waste products out of cells. It is also important in muscle function, helping to transmit messages between nerves and muscles, and is important to heart function.

A healthy kidney regulates potassium in the blood. If you consume potassium in excess from your diet or food additives, the kidney removes it from the blood and it is excreted as waste in your urine. As kidney function declines this function may be imperfect and some potassium can remain in the blood. The culprit of excess potassium may be food additives and medication. We will learn more about this shortly.

Guidelines for Potassium In the Diet

The recommended dietary allowance guideline for adults is 4,700 mg per day for healthy adults.

A low potassium diet recommends 2350 mg potassium per day (60 meq) *Following a low potassium diet when your potassium is normal does not improve kidney health.* Quite the opposite you might be depriving yourself of valuable nutrients which might contribute to an alkaline environment. I tried to keep most of the recipes in this book under 600 mg potassium to make them useful for most stages of chronic kidney disease.

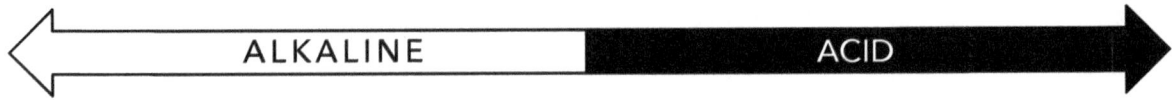

Convenience Food and Excessive Potassium

When we consider potassium sources in our diet we usually think fruits and vegetables. While that is partially correct, huge contributors of potassium are food additives founds in fast food and processed food. Read labels on packaged food and you will come across potassium tripolyphosphate, tetrapotasium phosphate. These flavor enhancers, shelf life extenders are in most packaged products. *These chemicals are very efficiently absorbed and are a very significant cause of elevated potassium levels in the blood.*

Compare potassium content of processed food to non-processed food

WISE potato chips 1150 mg	Fast Food French fries 584 mg	1/2 Baked Potato 450 mg

3 oz Fast Food hamburger 2114 mg	or	3 oz hamburger no additives 397 mg

Fast Food chicken 1210 mg potassium	or	6 oz fresh chicken 624 mg potassium

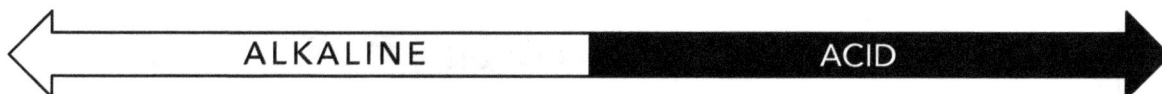

ALKALINE | ACID

Comparing Animal-Based Foods and Plant Based Food for Potassium Content

Food item	Potassium in miligrams
4 oz Fish	450 mg
4 oz chicken	416 mg
4 oz beef	422 mg
½ cup lentil	498 mg
½ cup kidney beans	360 mg

By substituting legumes and beans for animal protein, you are substituting equivalent potassium items for another.

Eating more vegetables and fruits might stabilize potassium in your blood. Research has shown that when we consume animal protein, which promotes an acidic environment, it prompts potassium to leave the cells and travel outside the cell into the blood stream. Shifting intracellular potassium to extracellular space.

> **An alkaline environment keeps potassium inside the cell preventing hyperkalemia (high potassium)**
>
> **Acidic environment causes potassium to leave the cell causing hyperkalemia**

Medications and Potassium

Some medications also may promote higher potassium levels. One class are the NSAIDS. Non-steroidal anti-inflammatory drugs, some common ones are; Celebrex, ibuprofen and naproxen.

Other medications such as: Amiloride, a sodium channel blocker, Spironolactone, Cyclosporine, Tacrolimus, Tremetoprim, Pentamidine, Beta blockers, Succinylcholine, Digoxin.

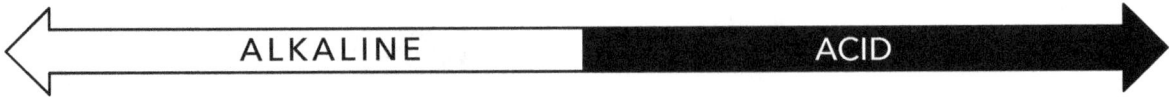

Other "Non-Dietary" Causes of Hyperkalemia

Medications known as ACE inhibitors and ARB's are used due to their protective effect on kidney, especially in the presence of diabetes. They are "potassium sparing" keeping the potassium in the blood rather than excreting it in the urine. Doctors try to use the medications as much as possible due to their positive effect on kidney health.

Laboratory Tests for Measuring Potassium Levels In Your Blood

An acceptable potassium level is normally 3.6-5.1 millimoles per liter (mmol/L)
There may be some small difference between different laboratories.

Defining Hyperkalemia Using Laboratory Values

Hyperkalemia is the medical term that describes a potassium level in your blood that's higher than normal. Always be aware of your most recent potassium lab test, here are some guidelines from the National Kidney Foundation.

If it is 3.5-5.0 . . . . .You are in the **SAFE** zone

If it is 5.1-6.0 . . . . .You are in the **CAUTION** zone

If it is higher than 6.0 . . . . .You are in the **DANGER** zone

Know Your Number

Please know your potassium number. Be an empowered patient who always requests his/hers labs and has a basis for comparison. If you happen to be constipated the day of the lab draw, this may give you a high potassium reading. However, if you are following my alkaline diet, consuming lots of vegetables, fruit, whole grain and legumes, a high fiber diet will promote very regular bowel movements.

I seldom see a CKD stage 1-4 patient with a potassium level much greater than the mild range. In Stage 5 *pre-dialysis* it can be more common.

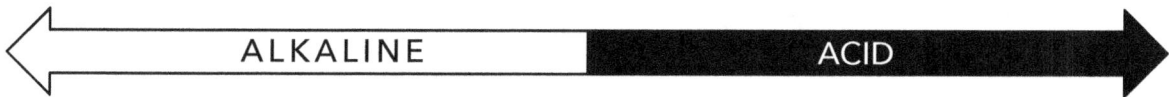

In Dr. Wessen's study following patients for 3 years, potassium levels stayed well within the acceptable limits by following a healthy alkaline diet.

Medications to Lower Potassium

There are medications that bind potassium if needed. One has been around for a long time, Kayexalate (sodium polystyrene sulfonatate). A newer medication approved by the FDA in 2015, Patiromer, trade name Veltassa. I have found that physicians vary quite a bit in their use of these potassium lowering medications. Some doctors use them routinely others very sparingly, seems to be a professional choice.

CHAPTER 8

All About Phosphorus

Phosphorus is an essential mineral primarily used for growth and repair of body cell and tissues. All body cells contain phosphorus, with 85% found in bones and teeth.

Normal working kidneys can remove extra phosphorus from the blood. As a patient progresses through the stages of chronic kidney disease, the kidneys may not be able to keep up with the removal of excessive phosphorus intake. This excess phosphorus in the blood can pull calcium out of bones and deposit it in blood vessels, including vessels of the heart, lungs and soft tissue.

There have been some studies that found that higher laboratory values of phosphorus are associated with a more rapid decline of kidney function. *Keeping your phosphorus in the acceptable range is one of the tools which will slow progression of CKD.*

Normal Phosphorus Range

Lab values for phosphorus- normal range is 2.5-4.5 mg/dl

A Recommended Dietary Allowance for Phosphorus

In healthy individuals is 700-1200 mg per day. This is totally possible if your diet is mostly fresh, whole foods rather than processed food or fast food. There are estimates that a typical Western diet, with the addition artificial phosphates used for improving the taste and texture of processed meats, snack foods and beverages can easily add 300-500 mg of phosphorus per day.

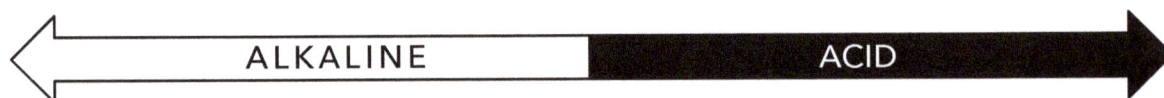

Strategies to Lower Phosphorus In the Plasma:

- restrict phosphorus intake to natural sources eat unprocessed whole food.

- keep to a minimum phosphorus from preservatives and flavor enhancers.

- keep animal protein intake to a reasonable portion size

> **To keep your phosphorus consumption down**
>
> **select fresh, unprocessed foods, preservative free foods. Plant based phosphorus is not well absorbed while artificial or chemically added phosphorus is extremely well absorbed**

Bioavailability of Different Sources of Phosphorus

Not all phosphorus is created equal. Plant based phosphorus is not well absorbed while artificial or chemically added phosphorus is extremely well absorbed.

Plant Based Phosphorus

Phosphorus found is whole wheat, nuts, lentils, grains and legumes is poorly absorbed. Only 10-30% is bioavailable and absorbed into the blood stream.

Animal Based Phosphorus

Phosphorus contained in dairy products; milk, cheese, yogurt, eggs, beef, chicken, turkey and fish is more bioavailable and absorbed at approximately 60-80%.

ALKALINE   ACID

Inorganic or preservative based phosphorus- Phosphorus is the main component of many preservatives and additive salts found in processed foods. Additives are used in food processing for a variety of reasons; extend shelf life, improve color, enhance flavor, and retain moisture. Common sources of inorganic phosphorus include certain beverages, enhanced or restructured meats, frozen meals, cereals, snack bars, processed or spreadable cheeses, instant products, and refrigerated bakery products. *It is believed that >90% of inorganic phosphorus may be absorbed in the intestinal tract, as compared to only 40 to 60% of the organic phosphorus present in natural food.*

> **phosphorus naturally found in beans, grains, legumes and seeds is not well absorbed by the body, less than 50% of phosphorus is absorbed**

> **Artificial phosphorus added to soft drinks, and processed foods is very well absorbed, more than 90% of the phosphorus is absorbed**

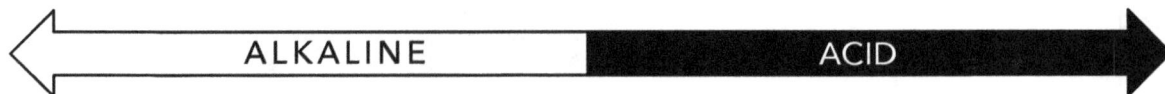

Common Phosphorus Salts Used in Food Processing

Product	Function	Phosphate Salt
Imitation cheese, buttermilk	texturizer	Disodium phosphate
Sport drink, whole egg product	emulsifier	Monosodium phosphate
Poultry product (cold cuts, fast food chicken)	moisture retention	Potassium tripolyphosphate
French fries, instant mashed potatoes	color	Sodium acid pyrophasphate
Frozen fish fillet	reduce purge, emulsfier	Sodium hexametaphosphate
Instant noodles, low sodium meats	flavor enhancer	Sodium tripplyphosphate
Sausage and deli meats	moisture retention	Tetrasodium pyrophosphate
Cheese	antimicrobial	Trisodium triphosphate

Common Beverages Contain Added Phosphorus Salts

AMP Energy

Aquafina Flavorsplash

Coka-Cola and Pepsi-Cola all forms regular and diet

Fanta Orange, Red Tangerine

Fruit works all flavors

Gatorade and G2 all flavors

Hawaiian Punch all flavors

Lipton Brisk Tea- green, lemon, raspberry, sweet tea, no calorie lemon, all plastic bottled teas, sparkling tea.

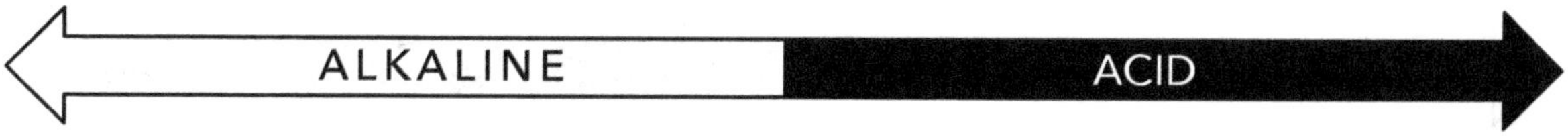
ALKALINE
ACID

Nestea diet lemon, green tea citrus, diet green tea, red tea pomegranate passion, raspberry

Mountain Dew code red

Mr. Pibb Xtra, Zero, Dr. Pepper

Propel water- all flavors

Tropicana Fruit Drinks all flavors

Compare Phosphorus Contenet of Processed Foods to Similar Fresh Foods

Chicken

KFC chicken breast 389 mg	or	3 oz Fresh chicken 190 mg
Tyson quick frozen with enhanced flavors added 317 mg	or	1 cup black beans 240 mg (absorbed 50%)

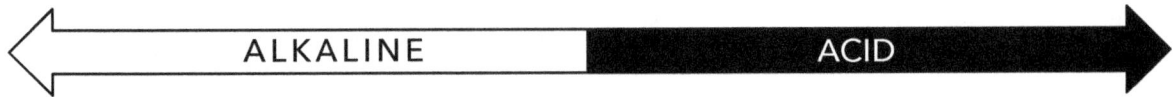

ALKALINE ← → **ACID**

Fish

Filet of fish 190 mg (contains only 1.5 oz actual fish mostly fillers and breading	or	3 oz Unprocessed Cod 190 mg

Breakfast

Fast Food Egg. cheese, sausage on a biscuit 664 mg	or	Homemade egg sandwich 190 mg

Beverages

No additive iced tea 0 mg phos	or	Water 0 mg phos
Lipton iced tea 100-189 mg phos	or	Hawaiian Punch 260 mg phos

In summary, by eating more fresh, whole food vs. processed food, the dietary phosphorus intake is much reduced. By consuming more plant-based protein vs. animal protein the phosphorus intake is further decreased and a more alkaline environment is created.

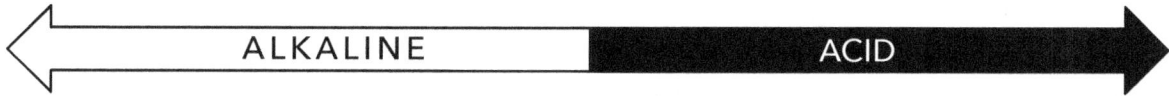

CHAPTER 9

The Benefit of Plant-Based Protein

The addition of plant based protein as a benefit of managing progression of CKD has been studied extensively. Some studies have shown that a 65% vegetarian diet reduced albuminurina (protein in the urine), urine urea nitrogen, and serum phosphorus levels. While a diet composed mostly of animal protein did not show these same results. Other studies showed that transitioning to a mostly plant-based diet improved glomerular filtration rates (GFR- the test used to measure kidney function) and proteinuria.

In my quest to promote an alkaline environment for best kidney health, I am suggesting replacing some animal protein with soy based protein. I want to address first how soy has shown to benefit progression of chronic kidney disease and secondly, I want to assure my readers of its safety.

There Is Evidence That Soy Protein Intake Has a Beneficial Effect on Kidney Function.

An analysis of 9 different studies looked at the benefit of adding soy protein to the diet and its effect on kidney function in chronic kidney disease.

The conclusion was positive in all the studies. There was a significant reduction in serum creatinine level indicating improved kidney function. In addition, there was also reduction in serum cholesterol, triglycerides and significant reduction in serum phosphorus levels.

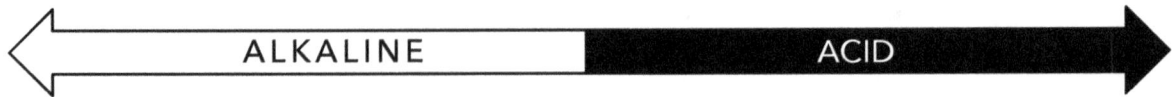

Research On the Benefits of Soy

Soy is available in a few different forms. It sold as tofu or bean curd, made by letting soy milk curdle and forming it into soft white blocks. The curds can be made into crumbles and are often flavored to make them recipe friendly.

Soy is also available in tablets, capsules and powders. According to the National Institutes of Health, National Center For Complementary and Integrative Health, soy is safe when consumed in normal dietary amounts. The most common side effects may be digestive upsets. Risk may be present when soy is consumed in pills, powders and extracts which contribute excessive amounts of the soy extract isoflavone. According to NIH, it is safe for women who have had breast cancer to eat soy food *in its* **natural state** *however the soy supplements and isoflavone extracts safety is uncertain.*

I would encourage you to consume soy as tofu rather than powders, capsules or additions to energy bars.

Plant Based Protein Sources

Animal protein contains approximately 8 grams of protein per ounce, a card size serving (3 oz) of animal protein provides 24 grams of protein.

How Much Protein Is Needed?

A usual recommendation is .8 grams of protein per kilogram of *ideal body weight.* If we try to follow a mostly plant-based diet the recommendations are 1.0 gram per kilogram of ideal body weigh

A deck of card portion of animal protein is a reasonable serving size. Larger quantity for fish since it is usually quite thin.

```
←————— ALKALINE | ACID —————→
```

Plant Based Protein Sources

Food	Protein Content
Edamame- cooked soybeans	18 grams in cup
Tempeh- fermented soy	16 grams in 3 oz
Tofu	12 grams in 3oz
Lentils	9 grams in ½ cup cooked
Quinoa	8 grams in 1 cup cooked
Black beans	7.5 grams in ½ cup cooked
Lima Beans	7.3 grams in ½ c cooked
Peanut butter	7 grams in 2 tablespoons
Wild rice	6.5 grams in 1 cup cooked
Chick Peas	7 grams in ½ cup cooked
Almonds	6 grams in ¼ cup
Chia Seeds	6 grams in 2 Tablespoons

Other Protein Sources

Food	Protein Content
Chicken, fish, red meat	8 grams in 1 oz
Egg	7 grams in 1 egg
Egg white	3.5 grams in 1 egg white
Cow milk	8 grams in 8 oz
Almond milk	1 gram in 8 oz
Soy milk	7 grams in 8 oz
Greek yogurt	10 grams in 8 oz

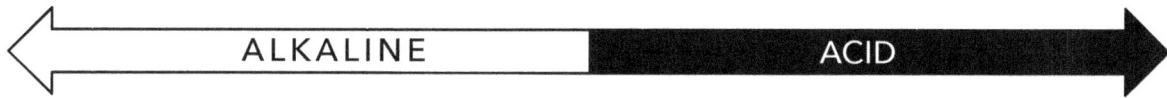

ALKALINE   ACID

CHAPTER 10

Meal Planning

Find Yourself In the Boxes Below

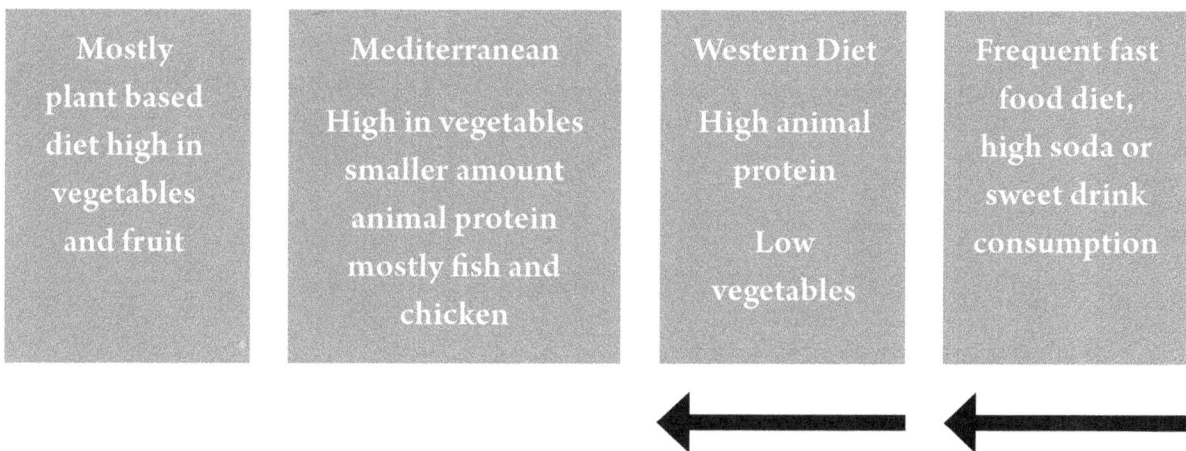

| Mostly plant based diet high in vegetables and fruit | Mediterranean

High in vegetables smaller amount animal protein mostly fish and chicken | Western Diet

High animal protein

Low vegetables | Frequent fast food diet, high soda or sweet drink consumption |

Can you commit to making some changes and moving over to a box on the left?

Human behavior takes time to change so try to set small goals and strategize a path to implement these goals.

Goals Month 1

- Give up all fructose sweetened drinks; soda, sweet tea, juice

- Dairy products: Reduce fat in milk to fat free or at least 1%

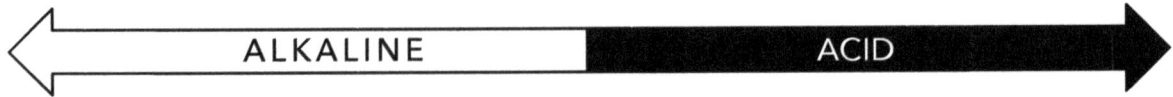

- Have your last fast food meal

- Reduce red meat to once per week

- Have a few plant based protein meals per week

- Have 1-2 cups of vegetables or salad with lunch and dinner

- Walk 10 minutes daily

Goals Month 2

- Increase walking or some type of activity to most days of the week

- Eat out at places which use only fresh, unprocessed ingredients

- Reduce animal protein meals to one per day

- Reduce red meat to one meal per month

Goals Month 3

Keep up with the changes you made in month 1 and 2.

Can you select one new goal for this month?

It takes a bit of time for the inflamation in your body to subside and for your labs to reflect the changes you have made. If you have protein in your urine, this will improve but I found it takes months not weeks.

Meal Planning

What you need to know: Your latest potassium lab number

Guidelines from the National Kidney Foundation.

If it is 3.5-5.0 . . . . .You are in the **SAFE** zone

If it is 5.1-6.0 . . . . .You are in the **CAUTION** zone

If it is higher than 6.0 . . . . .You are in the **DANGER** zone

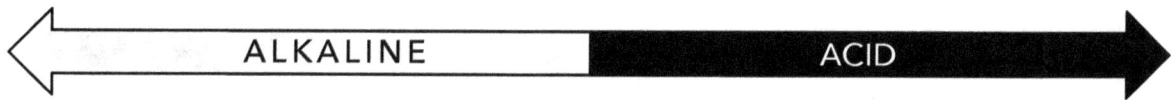

If your potassium number is between 3.5-5.0 you can pick **any** recipe and cereal.

If it is in the caution or danger zone please select low potassium cereal and select lower potassium recipes. I have added modification for lowering potassium levels in recipes which exceed 600 mg.

Phosphorus- in chronic kidney disease the best way to stay within a healthy phosphorus budget is to eat unprocessed foods.

Putting It All Together

I have attempted to inundate you with science with the hope of showing you how increasing vegetables and fruit and decreasing animal protein and processed food will benefit your kidneys. I know it's a lot of science to take in but the benefit to your kidneys will be huge. I should also include that I hope I also made a convincing case for giving up high fructose corn syrup sweetened beverages.

Planning Your Meals

Many of you may have seen the USDA plate; heaping with vegetables, a more modest serving of starch and a deck of card serving of animal protein.

Selecting Healthier Animal Protein Sources

Meal planning: For starters lets primarily pick fish and poultry most days of the week, red meat on special occasions.

Add more fresh fruit and vegetables to your diet and protein from legumes and soy.

> **Select fish and poultry most days of the week, red meat on special occasions.**

ALKALINE ← → ACID

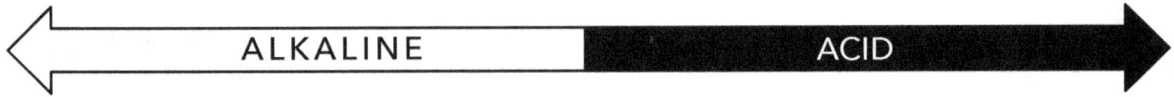

Balance the proportions of your plate

Plate Planner – Renal

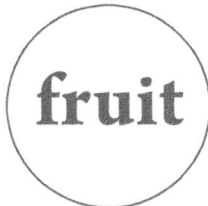

fruit
Fresh fruit, one piece or half cup

Chicken, fish, tofu, eggs, seafood

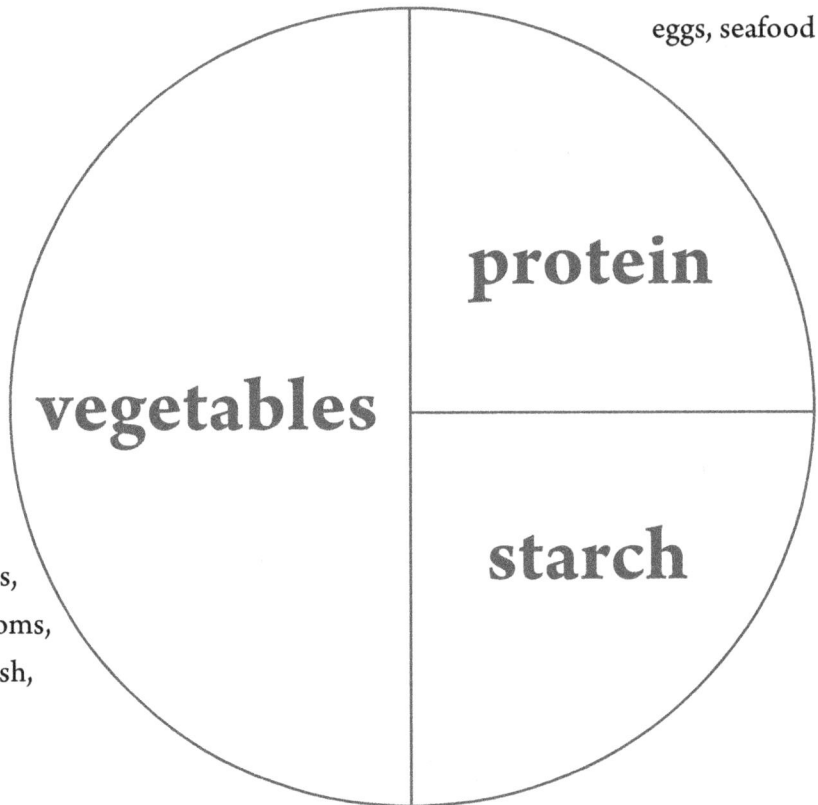

All non-starch vegetables are excellent. Asparagus, beets, broccoli, cabbage, cauliflower, carrots, eggplant, celery, cucumbers, green beans, leeks, iceberg lettuce, mushrooms, onions, radishes, pepper, squash, zucchini

vegetables

protein

starch

Brown rice, whole wheat pasta, corn, peas, lima beans, all dried beans (black, kidney, white) lentils, bulgur, quinoa, cous cous, potatoes

30 Days of Sample Meals

Day	Breakfast	Lunch	Snack	Dinner
1	Plain oatmeal with craisins, brown sugar, blueberries coffee	tuna sandwich carrots, grapes unsweetened iced tea with lemon and mint	apples 1 tsp peanut butter	Greek layered salad raspberries, cool whip, sparkling water
2	Frosted Mini wheats, cow milk or rice milk,1 tsp raisins strawberries	blueberry faro salad unsweetened lemonade	3 cups popcorn	unstuffed cabbage soup hearty bread sherbet
3	old fashioned Cheerios ½ banana	Kashi brand frozen entrée with salad and fruit	hummus and vegetables	Moroccan chicken Cous cous green beans
4	overnight oats coffee	additive free turkey sandwich, small garden salad, apple	pretzels and craisins	eggplant teriyaki stir fry
5	2 eggs, wheat toast, butter, all fruit spread	squash soup, whole grain crackers, apple slices	cheese stick and grapes	loaded potato skins with turkey, green salad with Italian olive oil dressing
6	Rice Krispies, cow milk or rice milk, sliced peaches	lemony white bean and arugula salad, sparkling water	3 cups popcorn	tilapia w Thai curry sauce, ½ c broccoli, chocolate cherry bar
7	avocado toast	minestrone soup with hearty bread	vegetables and guilt free ranch dip	chicken broccoli salad with buttermilk dressing
8	Greek yogurt with homemade muesli	green bean and tuna salad	rice cake, 2 T peanut butter	Mexican street corn tostada

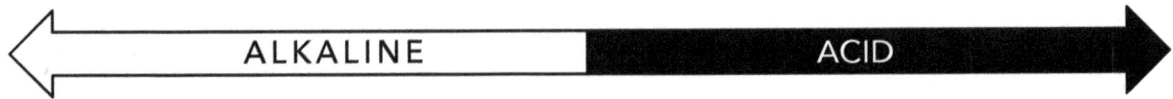

Day	Breakfast	Lunch	Snack	Dinner
9	Corn Flakes with berries, cow milk or rice milk	Amy's frozen meal	animal crackers	Moo Shoo chicken
10	morning smoothie	additive free turkey meat on whole wheat bread and side salad	hummus and vegetables	French chicken stew and hearty bread
11	2 eggs, whole wheat toast	Vietnamese chicken salad with rice noodles	3 cups popcorn	lime cous cous with vegetables
12	overnight oats	butternut squash soup	cheese stick and grapes	salmon bowl
13	Kashi Heart To Heart cereal with cow milk or rice milk	Eating Well frozen meal with chicken	vanilla wafers	General Tso Tofu serve with rice and veg of your choice
14	Greek yogurt with homemade muesli	greens and veg salad with frozen short cut additive free chicken strips, Paul Newman dressing	vegetables and guilt free ranch dip	black bean tacos
15	oatmeal with raisins and nut garnish	Eating Well frozen meal with chicken	pretzels and 1-2 oz cheese	roasted eggplant with tomatoes and mint
16	2 eggs whole grain toast and fruit	portabella mushroom burger	3 cups popcorn	fried cauliflower rice with chicken
17	morning smoothie	taco salad	vanilla wafers	baked spaghetti squash with shrimp

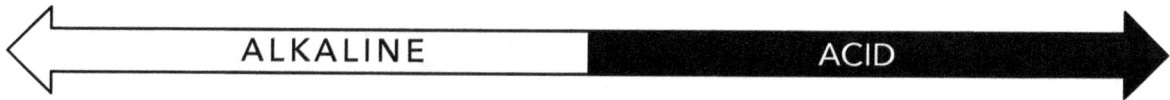

Day	Breakfast	Lunch	Snack	Dinner
18	Life cereal with berries	egg salad sandwich on whole wheat bread, raw veggies	snack hummus and vegetables	Korean grilled chicken served with rice and vegetable of your choice
19	overnight oats	lentil soup	apple and peanut butter	sheet pan fajitas
20	omelet with salmon and avocado	additive free turkey sandwich on whole grain bread, side baby carrots,	grapes and cheese stick	fish taco
21	Kashi Heart To Heart cereal with cow milk or rice milk	lentil apple walnut salad	vegetables and guilt free ranch dip	dijon salmon with green beans and rice pilaf
22	morning smoothie	tuna salad sandwich on whole grain bread side salad and fruit	½ c cottage cheese and fruit	stuffed portabella mushrooms
23	Greek yogurt with homemade muesli	Kashi brand frozen meal side salad and apple	hummus and vegetables	Greek shrimp barley salad
24	omelet with vegetables and whole grain toast	greens and veg salad with frozen short cut additive free chicken strips, Paul Newman dressing	pretzels and 1-2 oz cheese	Moroccan chicken served with rice and vegetable of your choice
25	Smart Pops with berries	black bean squash soup, corn tortillas, water	hummus and vegetables	orange maple salmon with orzo and vegetable of your choice

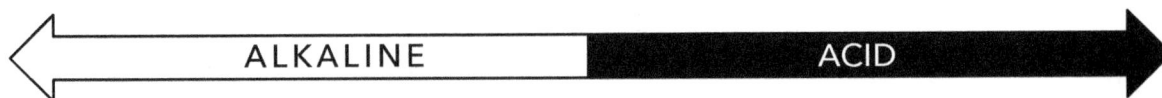

Day	Breakfast	Lunch	Snack	Dinner
26	unfrosted mini wheats, cow milk or rice milk and fruit	Smart Ones frozen entrees "Smart made with side salad and fresh fruit	3 cups popcorn	pesto cauliflower rice with shrimp
27	Greek yogurt with homemade muesli	additive free turkey sandwich on whole wheat bread	vegetables and guilt free ranch dip	black bean and butternut squash enchiladas
28	scrambled eggs whole grain English muffin and fruit	additive free turkey sandwich on whole grain bread, side salad and berries	½ c cottage cheese and fruit	Mexican quinoa salad served with garden salad and olive oil vinaigrette
29	morning smoothie	hearty tuscan soup with hearty bread	hummus and vegetables	Cuban chicken with coleslaw
30	Corn flakes cow milk or rice milk and craisins	Amy's Brand frozen entree	pretzels and 1-2 oz cheese	turmeric braised chicken with cauliflower served over rice or orzo

ALKALINE ACID

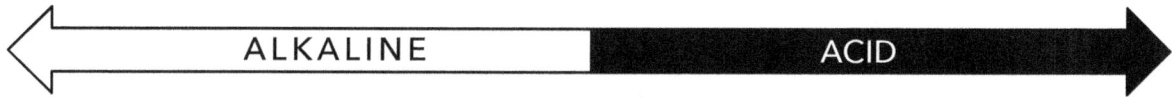

Cereal List A – Low to Moderate In Potassium Content

plain oatmeal	Cheerios	Rice Krispies
Apple Jacks	Special K	Kashi Heart to Heart
Smart Start	Corn Pops	Corn Flakes
Rice, Chex	Corn Chex	Life
Frosted or unfrosted Mini Wheats		

List B High Potassium Content – Limit These If Your Potassium Is 5.1 or Higher

Granola type	Raisin Bran	Wheat Bran
All Bran	Kashi Go Lean	
Muesli flavored quick oatmeal		

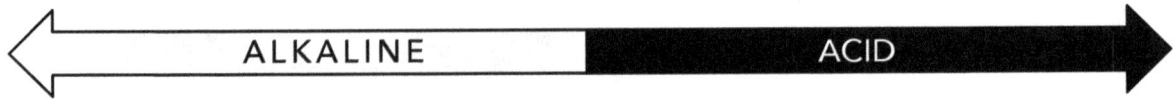

FRUIT CHOICES (source of natural potassium)

Serving is 1 piece fruit or ½ cup

Low	Medium	High
Daily Selection (less than 100 mg per serv	Twice a week (100-200 mg per serv) If your potassium is 5.1 or higher	Not recommended. More than 200 mg per serving If your potassium is 5.1 or higher
Apples and applesauce	Apricots	Dried apricots
Blackberries	Cantaloupe	Canned apricots
Blueberries	Cherries	Avocado
Shredded coconut	Clementine's	Banana
Pears	Craisins	Dates
Pineapple	Grapes	Figs
Raspberries	Mandarin oranges	Guava
Rhubarb	Mango	Kiwi
Strawberries	Papayas	Honeydew Melon
Watermelon	Plums	Prunes
	Tangerines	Raisins
	Canned peaches	Oranges
		Prune juice
		Orange juice

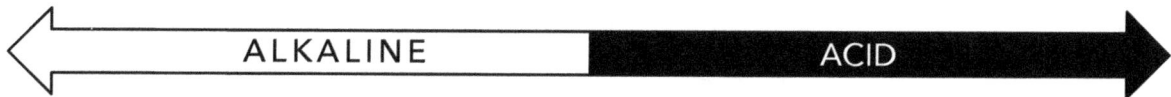

VEGETABLE CHOICES (source of natural potassium)
a serving is ½ c cooked or 1 c raw

Low	Medium	High
Daily Selection (less than 100 mg per serv)	Twice a week (100-200 mg per serv) If your potassium is 5.1 or higher	Not recommended. More than 200 mg per serving If your potassium is 5.1 or higher
Alfalfa sprouts	Asparagus	Artichoke
Green beans	Beets	Avocado
Wax beans	Broccoli	Bamboo shoots fresh
Carrots	Bok choy	Beet greens
Cucumber	Cabbage	Brussels sprouts
Corn	Cauliflower	Black eyed peas
Endive	Celery	Chard
Escarole	Collard Greens	Chinese cabbage
Iceberg lettuce	Eggplant	Kohlrabi
Green peas	Kale	Parsnip
Leeks	Lima beans	Potato
Red or orange pepper	Mushrooms	Pumpkin
2 slices of tomato	Okra	Pumpkin seeds
Onions as garnish	Onions as meal	Rutabaga
Spaghetti squash	Green peppers	Sauerkraut
Water Chestnuts canned	Radish	Soy beans
Watercress	Summer squash	Spinach
	Soaked potatoes *	Sunflower seeds
	Snow peas	Water chestnuts fresh
	Turnips	Winter squash
		Tomato sauce

*To reduce potassium in a potato: peel, cut into cubes, soak covered in water overnight.

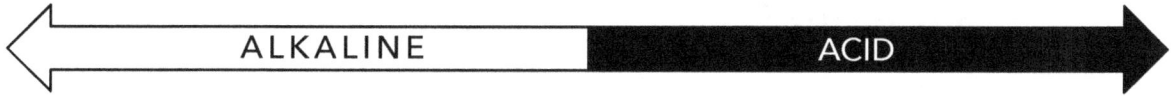

ALKALINE | ACID

CHAPTER 11

Breakfast Recipes

Overnight Strawberry and Cream Oats

Overnight Oats with Berries and Toasted Coconut

Homemade Muesli

Avocado Toast

Morning Smoothie

Omelet with Vegetables

Avocado and Salmon Omelet

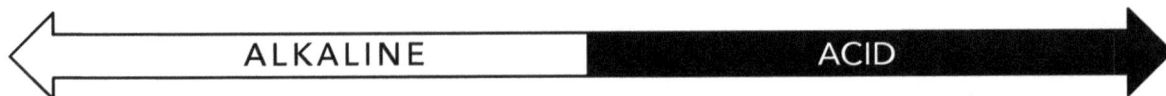

Overnight Strawberry and Cream Oats

SERVES 1

Ingredients

½   cup almond milk

⅓   cup steel oats

½   cup strawberries or any other berry

1   tsp chia seeds

2   tsp honey

Directions

1.   Combine all ingredients in a glass mason jar. Refrigerate overnight. Top with granola or crushed nuts.

This recipe can be modified to change the fruit, can add peanut butter, shredded coconut, nuts. Can use rice or soy milk instead of almond milk.

Nutrition per serving: calories 184, carbohydrates 33g, protein 5g, fat 4g, potassium 292 mg, phosphorus 170 mg, sodium 90 mg

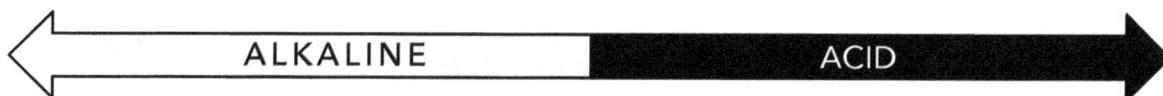

Overnight Oats with Berries and Toasted Coconut

Using Kefir adds 12 strains of active probiotic cultures
great for improving the GUT bacteria.

SERVES 2

Ingredients

1⅓   cup low fat kefir

⅔   cup old fashioned oats

2   tsp honey

¼   tsp ground cinnamon

½   cup blueberries

½   cup strawberries

2   T unsweetened coconut flakes- roasted

Directions

1. Combine first 4 ingredients in a bowl, cover and refrigerate overnight

2. Divide oat mixture between 2 bowls. Top with berries and coconut.

Nutrition per serving: calories 229, Carbohydrates 42g, protein 10g, fat 4g, potassium 400 mg, phosphorus 270 mg, sodium 229mg

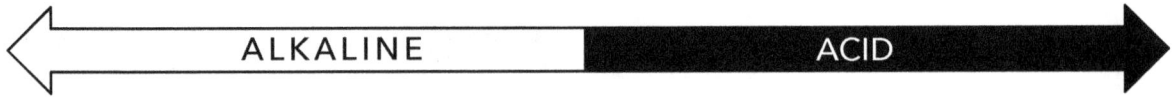

Homemade Muesli

MAKES 20 SERVINGS ½ CUP EACH

Ingredients

5	cups rolled oats
2	cups unsweetened shredded coconut
2	cups sliced almonds
½	cup flax seed
1	cup raisins

Directions

1. Mix all ingredients, store in airtight container- can store up to 1 month

2. To serve top with rice or almond milk and berries.

Nutrition per serving: calories 221, protein 6g, carbohydrate 20g, fat 11g, potassium 268 mg, phosphorus 173 mg

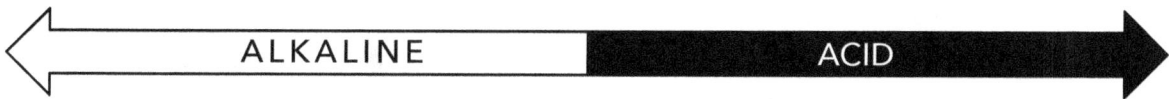

Avocado Toast

Ingredients

1   slice whole grain bread

¼th   medium avocado

1   teaspoon lemon juice

        pepper to taste

Directions

1. Scoop flesh from avocado into a bowl.

2. Add lemon juice and pepper mix well and mash gently

3. Toast bread, top with avocado, season to taste and serve.

Nutrition per serving: calories 125, carbohydrates 15, protein 4g, fat 6g, potassium 236mg, phosphorus 77 mg, sodium 130 mg

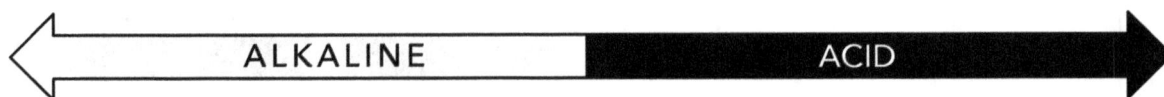

Morning Smoothie

SERVES 1

Ingredients

1   cup frozen berries

1   cup frozen peaches

½   cup tofu

1   cup almond milk

Directions

1. Mix all ingredients in a blender until well combined.

Nutrition per serving: calories 129, protein 6g, carbohydrates 23g, potassium 261mg, phosphorus 72 mg

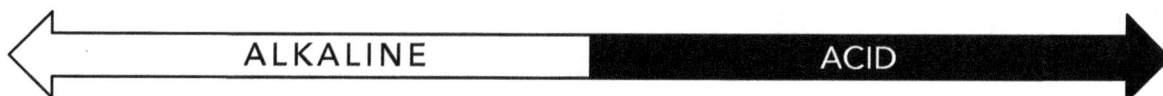

Omelet with Vegetables

SERVES 1

Ingredients

¼   cup frozen corn

⅓   cup zucchini

3   tbs green onions

2   T water

¼   tsp Mrs. Dash

     Black pepper to taste

2   large egg whites

1   large egg

1   oz cheddar cheese

Directions

1. Heat a pan over medium heat. Coat pan with cooking spray.

2. Add corn, zucchini and onions to pan. Sauté for 4 minutes or until vegetables are tender. Remove from heat

3. In a bowl combine egg, egg whites, pepper and Mrs. Dash in a bowl stirring well.

4. Place pan over medium heat, add cooking spray. Pour egg mixture into pan, cook until the edges begin to set about 2-3 minutes. Lift the edges of the omelet with a spatula and let the runny egg mixture flow.

5. Spoon the vegetable mixture onto half the omelet, sprinkle cheese over the vegetable mixture.

6. Fold the omelet in half cook 1 minute or until the cheese melts.

Nutrition per serving: calories 187, protein 22g, carbohydrates 12g, fat 6g, potassium 352 mg, Phosphorus 218 mg, sodium 270 mg

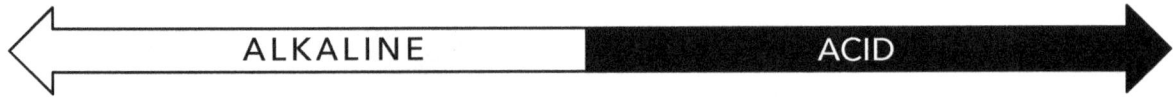

Avocado and Salmon Omelet

SERVES 1

A healthy breakfast rich in protein, Omega 3 and healthy fats. The current recommendations are for 5 whole eggs per week. If you love this and want it often I suggest using 1 egg white and 1 whole egg to reduce cholesterol.

Ingredients

2	eggs
1	tsp milk
1	tsp olive oil
¼	medium avocado sliced
1	oz smoked salmon or "lox"
1	T basil- fresh, chopped

Directions

1. Beat the eggs with milk in a small bowl

2. Heat 1 tsp oil in a nonstick skillet. Add the egg mixture and cook until the bottom is set but the center is a bit runny. Flip the omelet and cook 30 seconds to 1 min more.

3. Transfer to a plate, top with salmon, avocado and basil. Fold over and serve

Makes 1 omelet.

Nutrition per serving: calories 260, protein 20g, carbohydrates 3g, fat 18g, (mostly healthy monosaturated fat) potassium 374mg, phosphorus 305 mg, sodium 246mg.

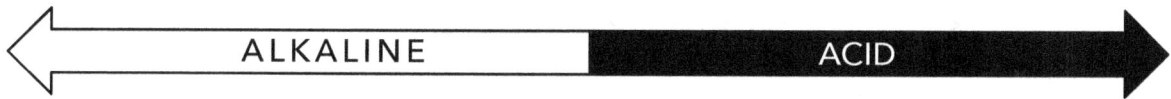

ALKALINE   ACID

CHAPTER 12

Soups and Stews

French Chicken Stew

Lentil Soup

Black Bean and Squash Soup

Lemon Chicken Tortellini Soup

Hearty Tuscan Soup

Minestrone Soup

Grandma's Chicken Noodle Soup

Butternut Squash Soup

Unstuffed Cabbage Soup with Ground Turkey

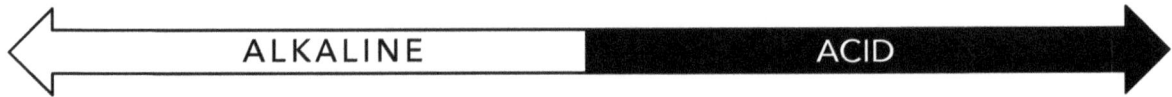

French Chicken Stew

This is one of my all-time favorite stews, the rich fragrance and
hearty taste will make it one of yours too.

SERVES 6 (1 CUP SERVINGS)

Ingredients

3   T purpose flour- divided

2   lb boneless chicken breast cut into 1 inch cubes

2½   T olive oil (divided)

2   med carrots chopped

2   med celery stalks chopped

1   large onion chopped

3   garlic cloves minced

2   cups dry white wine

1½   cups low fat reduced sodium chicken broth- use home made or additive free broth

1   T tomato paste

1   T fresh thyme chopped

2   bay leaves

8   oz pearl onion frozen (thawed)

8   oz (3 cups) brown mushrooms) sliced

Directions

1.   Add 2 T of the flour to a large bowl. Add the chicken and toss to coat.

2.   Heat 1 T oil in a pan over medium heat. Add the chicken in batches, don't over crowd, sauté until well browned. Turn every couple of minutes. Remove the chicken and set aside.

3.   Add another 1T of oil, add carrots, celery, and onion cook until browned for 8 minutes. Add the garlic and sauté for 1 minute. Add the remaining flour, mix to coat the vegetables. Cook I minute.

4.   Add the wine, bring to a boil, reduce heat and cook 5-7 minutes, stirring often.

5.   Add the chicken broth, tomato paste, thyme and bay leaves. Add the chicken, reduce heat to low and simmer covered for 40 minutes.

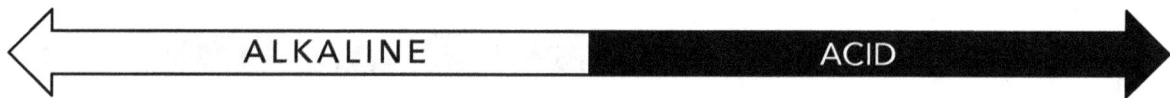

6.   While the chicken is simmering. Add ½ T oil to pan, cook the pearl onion and mushrooms until they are brown 6-8 minutes.

7.   Remove bay leaves from the soup add the onions and mushrooms. Simmer uncovered for 5-7 minutes. Season with pepper, garnish with parsley and serve.

Nutrition per serving: calories 265, carbohydrates 14g, protein 31g, fat 8g, potassium 565 mg, phosphorus 270 mg, sodium 225 mg

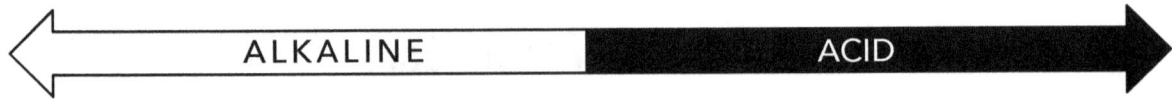

Lentil Soup

SERVES 4 (1⅓ CUP)

Ingredients

1	tsp olive oil
¾	cup chopped scallions
2	garlic cloves minced
1	medium tomato chopped or can use canned low sodium chopped tomatoes
¼	cup fresh cilantro chopped
1	tsp cumin powder
1	cup dried lentils
½	cup brown rice- uncooked
4	cups low sodium chicken broth or vegetable broth
1	bay leaf
	Black pepper to taste
1	tsp salt
	Garnish: Sour cream, scallions

Directions

1. Heat a large pot over medium heat. Add oil, scallions, garlic and tomato. Season with pepper. Cook stirring for 10 minutes.

2. Stir in ¼ cup chopped cilantro and cumin stir for 1 minute

3. Add lentils, rice, broth and bay leaf. Bring to a boil, reduce heat to medium low, cover and cook for 30 minutes. Check on the lentils, cook till soft.

4. Remove the bay leaf, using an immersion blender puree the soup. If you don't have one. Use blender, blend in 2- batches, don't fill blender to top (hot soups explode)

5. Taste soup, adjust seasonings

6. Serve garnished with sour cream, scallions and cilantro.

ALKALINE → ACID

Nutrition per serving: calories 188, carbohydrates 32g, protein 13g, fat 2g, potassium 599 mg, phosphorus 230 mg, sodium 460mg.

If your potassium is elevated (higher than 5.1) reduce the lentils to ¾ cup and increase brown rice. This will reduce the potassium to just over 500 mg which is considered a moderate potassium meal.

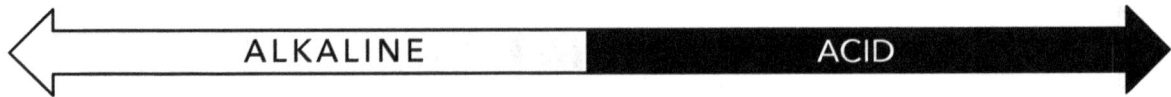

Black Bean and Squash Soup

This is a higher potassium meal. To reduce the potassium, double the squash and decrease the black beans to just 1 can. This will reduce the potassium to 373 mg per serving. I also recommend this be part of a vegetarian meal so you are not adding another potassium source from animal protein.

SERVES 7

Ingredients

2   cans black beans (you can reduce sodium by using dried beans)

5   cloves garlic peeled

1½   lb butternut squash (short cut –purchase squash already cut up)

1   T olive oil

1   yellow onion chopped

1   bay leaf

1   medium carrot chopped

1   celery stalk chopped

1   T ground cumin

1   jalapeno pepper, seeds removed, minced

7   cups homemade or store bough lower sodium vegetable broth

2   T lemon juice

Directions

1. If using whole squash, cut in half and bake in 400 F oven for 45 minutes. Let cool and scoop out the inside. If purchased already cut squash bake 30 minutes or until tender.

2. Heat olive oil in a large skillet, add onion, bay leaf and sauté for 5 minutes until soft and golden. Remove the bay leaf.

3. Add the beans (save ½ cup), carrot, celery, and jalapeno. Simmer for 15 minutes or until vegetables are tender.

4. Add the roasted squash, onion, cumin and vegetable broth. Cook 5 minutes

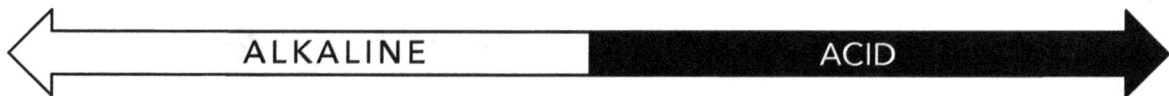

5. Allow soup to cool, using an immersion blender puree until its mostly smooth. Add the reserved ½ cup of beans and lemon juice.

6. Serve with warm tortillas

Nutrition per serving: calories 197, carbohydrates 35g, protein 11g, fat 2g, *potassium 681 mg, phosphorus, sodium 389 mgs

* If your potassium is above 5.1 decrease beans and increase the squash to reduce potassium to 373 mg. See modification at the beginning if the recipe.

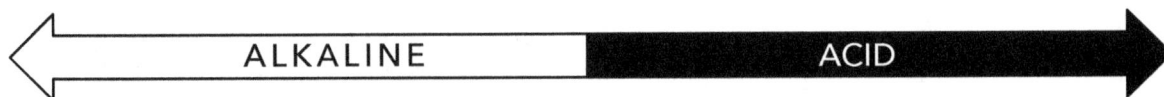

Lemon Chicken Tortellini Soup

This can be a versatile recipe, for a main meal soup add more chicken.
For a more traditional chicken soup can skip the lemon juice.

SERVES 6

Ingredients

1	T olive oil
½	cup yellow onion chopped
2	cloves garlic chopped
¾	cup carrots chopped
½	cup chopped celery
5	cup chicken broth- make your own or buy store bough, organic additive free lower in sodium
1½	tsp dried thyme
9	oz store bought tortellini filled with chicken or cheese
2	raw chicken breasts, cut into 1 inch cubes
5	oz fresh spinach
¼	cup lemon juice
2	T lemon zest

Directions

1. In a large Dutch oven or soup pot, heat olive oil over medium heat. Add onion and cook for 3 minutes. Add garlic, carrots and celery, cook additional 3 minutes.

2. Add chicken broth and thyme, bring to a boil.

3. Add the chicken, cook for 15 minutes

4. Add tortellini and cook according to package directions.

5. When the tortellini is almost done add the spinach cook for 1 minute

6. Remove from the heat, add lemon juice and lemon zest. Taste and adjust seasoning.

Nutrition per serving: calories 277, protein 19g, carbohydrates 38g, fat 6g, potassium 423mg, phosphorus 198 mg, sodium 470 mg

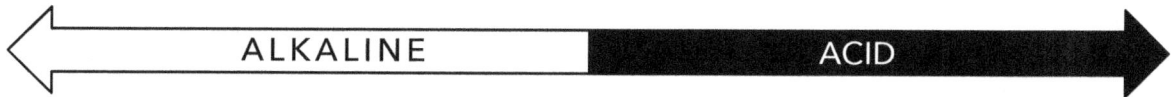

Hearty Tuscan Soup

Short cut tip: Many grocery stores, including Trader Joe's sell "mirepoix" already diced onions, celery and carrots. These save you lots of time in the kitchen and adds fabulous flavor.

You can individualize this soup by adding green beans, cauliflower or any vegetable you like. You can also add small shaped pasta

SERVES 8

Ingredients

8   cups low sodium chicken broth- make your own or buy organic, additive free broth.

3   garlic cloves minced

1   cup water

½   cup chopped onions

½   cup chopped celery

½   cup chopped carrots

1   cans navy beans, well rinsed

1   can 14 oz diced tomatoes

1   cup fresh spinach

2   cups few day old hearty bread torn into chunks

1   cup fresh basil

1   parmesan rind- I find these in the cheese section or ask for it at the counter (a secret weapon for soups)

½   cup grated parmesan cheese

Directions

1. Heat a large pot over medium heat, add olive oil, add garlic, onions, carrots and celery.

2. Stir in the broth, water, beans, tomatoes and parmesan rind. Bring to a boil, reduce heat and simmer for 30 minutes.

3. Using an immersion blender, blend until coarsely pureed, leaving some chunks.

4. At this step you can add your own individual vegetables or small pasta shapes. For vegetables cook 5 minutes or until almost done. For pasta 8-12 minutes or almost done.

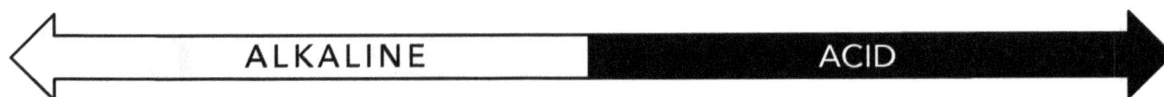

5. Stir in fresh spinach, cook 1 minute

6. Adjust seasoning

7. Add more broth is desired thinner soup

8. Ladle into bowls top with fresh basil, bread chunks and parmesan cheese.

Nutrition per serving: calories 170, carbohydrates 18g, protein 10g, fat 3g, potassium 465 mg, phosphorus 151mg, sodium 490 mg

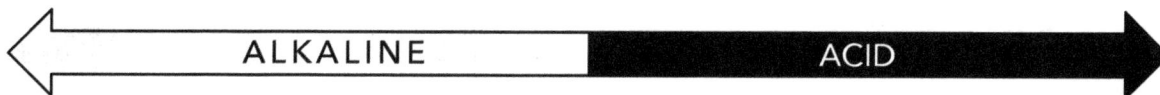

Minestrone Soup

SERVES 8

Adding a Parmesan rind to soups gives it a rich flavor you can add to any soup recipe. They are usually on sale in the gourmet cheese section.

Ingredients

1	15 oz can of white beans, drained and rinsed			
4	cups- divided homemade chicken broth or store bought additive free low sodium			
2	tsp olive oil	½	cup chopped onion
1	cup diced carrots	½	cup diced celery
2	garlic cloves minced	1	14 oz can of diced tomatoes
1	Parmesan rind	1	Fresh rosemary sprig
2	bay leaves	2	T chopped fresh basil
¼	cup chopped fresh parsley		Black pepper to taste
1	med zucchini diced		
2	cups cooked small pasta in desired shape		
	Garnish parmesan cheese		

Directions

1. Puree beans with 1 cup of broth in a blender or using an immersion blender set aside. If you like a more chunky soup you can set aside half of the beans and add later, to add texture.

2. Heat oil in a large pot over medium heat. Add the carrots, celery, onion garlic and sauté for 15 minutes

3. Add remaining broth, tomatoes, pureed beans, parmesan cheese rind, pepper, rosemary, basil and parsley. Bring to a boil, reduce heat, cover reduce heat to low and cook 40 minutes.

4. Add zucchini cook for additional 3 minutes

5. Cook pasta separately according to package directions.

6. Remove rosemary sprig, bay leaf.

7. Ladle soup into bowl, add ¼ c cooked pasta, sprinkle with parmesan cheese

Nutrition per serving: 216 calories, protein 11g, carbohydrates 38g, fat 3g, potassium 554 mg, phosphorus 150 mg, sodium 169 mg.

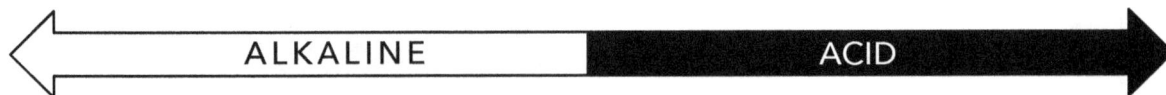

Grandma's Chicken Noodle Soup

SERVES 8

Ingredients

2   lbs chicken pieces (I found improved flavor using organic chicken bone-in combination of breast, leg and thigh)

1   whole onion peeled, cut into large chunks

2   medium carrots chopped

2   celery ribs chopped

2   garlic cloves chopped

3   bay leaves

¼   tsp black pepper

½   tsp thyme

¾   tsp salt

7   cups water

6   oz uncooked, dry pasta

½   cup dill chopped

Directions

1. In a large pot add chicken, whole peeled onion, carrot, celery, garlic, bay leaves, pepper, salt and COLD water. Cover and cook for 1 hour. Leave cover slightly ajar to let steam escape.

2. Remove foam on top, discard bay leaves. Remove the chicken and the bay leaves

3. Add pasta, cover and cook for 10 minutes or until pasta is ready

4. Shred the chicken with 2 forks, add chicken back to pot, add dill, heat 2-3 minutes and serve

Nutrition per serving: Calories 209, Protein 19g, Carbohydrates 19g, Fat 6g, Potassium 247 mg, Phosphorus 167mg, Sodium 505 mg

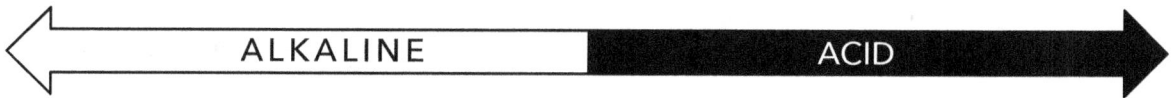

Butternut Squash Soup

SERVES 6

Nothing says fall like butternut squash soup. This is one of my favorite soups
and the entire family asks for it as soon as the days get colder.

Ingredients

1	large onion chopped
2	T butter
6	cups cubed butternut squash (I buy the short cut already peeled and chopped squash)
3	cups low sodium chicken broth- make your own or buy organic low sodium.
½	tsp dried marjoram
	Black pepper to taste
⅛	tsp cayenne pepper
½	of 8 oz pkg cream cheese- low fat
	Optional cinnamon and nutmeg

Directions

1. In a large saucepan sauté onions in butter until tender. Add squash, chicken broth, marjoram, black pepper and cayenne pepper. Bring to a boil, reduce heat, and simmer until squash is tender 20-30 min.

2. Using an immersion blender puree soup, add cream cheese, puree again. Do not let it come to a boil.

3. Serve- optional sprinkle of cinnamon or nutmeg, sometimes I have added a small amount of curry

Nutrition per serving: calories 162, protein 6g, carbohydrates 21g, fat 8g, potassium 561 mg, phosphorus 117 mg, sodium 111mg

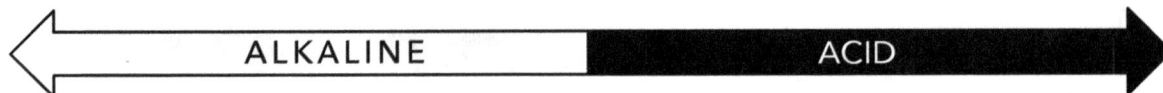

Unstuffed Cabbage Soup with Ground Turkey

This is a main meal soup meant to take the place of an entrée not as an appetizer to a main meal.

SERVES 8

Ingredients

1	Onion large diced
2	lb head cabbage cored and diced
1	4oz can tomato sauce
28	oz can peeled tomatoes with their juice
1	cup water
1	lb ground turkey
½	cup raw white rice
	Garnish- sour cream

Directions

1. In a large heavy pot combine onions, cabbage, tomato sauce, peeled tomatoes with their juice, water.

2. Bring to a boil, add ground turkey, reduce heat and simmer over low heat for 2 hours.

3. Remove the lid, add rice cook uncovered for additional 30 minutes.

4. I like to thicken the soup at this point- either remove 1 cup and puree in a blender and return to pot or I like to pass through with an immersion blender a few times. If you like a thinner consistency add water or low sodium broth.

5. Serve with a dollop of sour cream

Nutrition per serving: calories 191, protein 19g, carbohydrates 19g, fat 5g, potassium 559 mg, phosphorus 208 mg, sodium 570 mg

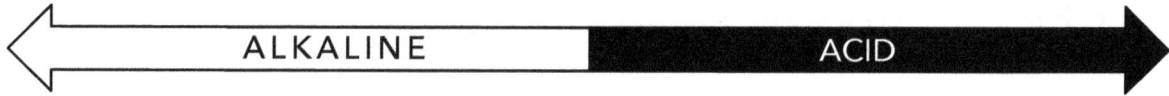

CHAPTER 13

Main Course Salads

(v- vegetarian, plant based protein)

Chicken Broccoli Salad with Buttermilk Dressing

Vietnamese Chicken Salad with Rice Noodles

Strawberry Chicken Salad with Feta

Green Bean Tuna Salad with Artichoke Hearts

Greek Shrimp and Barley Salad

Blueberry Faro Salad- v

Taco Salad- v

Mexican Style Quinoa Salad-v

Greek Salad Layered Over Hummus and Pita –v

Lemony White Bean and Arugula Salad-v

Lentil, Apple, and Walnut Salad with Apple Cider Dressing-v

Guilt Free Ranch Dressing with Assorted Vegetables

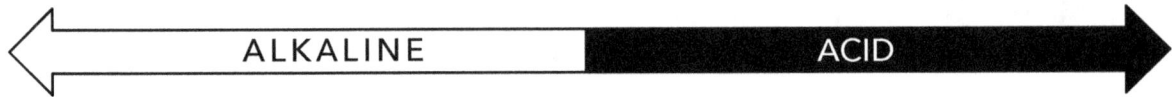

Chicken Broccoli Salad with Buttermilk Dressing

SERVES 4

This is a great weeknight recipe using some short cut ingredients.

Ingredients

3 cups broccoli coleslaw mix found in the produce section

2 cups chopped cooked chicken breast (use your own cooked chicken, or frozen chicken breast cooked per package directions or rotisserie chicken)

½ cup dried cherries

⅓ cup sliced celery

¼ cup chopped red onion

⅓ cup buttermilk

⅓ cup light mayonnaise

1 T honey

1 tsp dried mustard

4 cups baby spinach

Directions

1. Combine broccoli coleslaw mix, shredded chicken, dried cherries, celery, chopped red onion, toss

2. In a separate bowl, combine buttermilk, mayonnaise, honey, dried mustard, mix well

3. Add buttermilk mixture to broccoli mixture and combine well.

4. To serve place 1 cup baby spinach (or iceberg lettuce if potassium is above 5.1) top with ¼ chicken broccoli mixture

Nutrition per serving: calories 258, carbohydrates 27g, protein 23g, fat 7g, *potassium 590 mg, phosphorus 215 mg sodium 490mg

*(if your potassium is above 5.1 substitute iceberg lettuce for the raw spinach this will reduce the potassium to 480 mg)

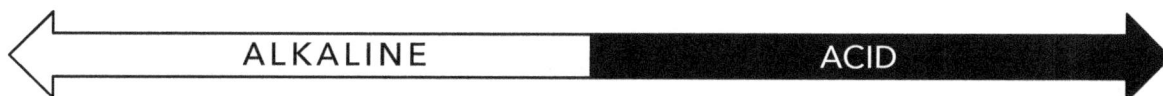

Vietnamese Chicken Salad with Rice Noodles

SERVES 4-6

Ingredients

For the dressing

3	serrano peppers- finely chopped, leave out the seeds unless you love SPICE
4	cloves garlic – chopped
2	T rice vinegar
2	T brown sugar
2	T fish sauce
6	T lime juice
6	T canola oil

For the salad

1	lb boneless chicken breast
6	oz rice noodles- you can buy the very thin ones or use thicker ones, you choose.
1	package shredded cabbage mixture or a small head of cabbage shredded
4	large carrots peeled and shredded or cut into slender 1 in matchsticks.

Garnish: cilantro, mint leaves, basil leaves, green onions

Directions for the dressing:

1. Thinly slice the serrano peppers and set aside

2. In a bowl add garlic, rice vinegar, brown sugar, fish sauce, lime juice, canola oil, serrano peppers. Whisk well in a bowl with a fork or wire whisk.

Chicken

3. Bring a pot of water to boil. Add the chicken, and simmer for 10 minutes. Turn off the heat and let the chicken sit (with lid on the pot) for another 20 minutes. Remove the chicken, let it cool.

4. Shred with 2 forks, drizzle with some of the prepared dressing to give it flavor.

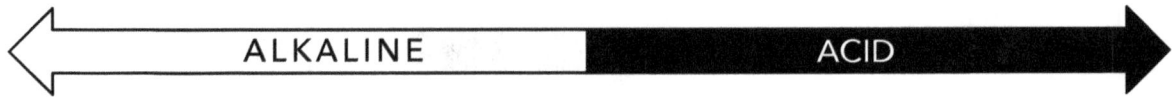

Noodles

5. Soak the noodles in a large bowl of cold water for 15 minutes until softened

6. Heat noodles in a small amount of dressing in a large skillet over high heat for about 5 minutes to give them flavor and crunch.

Salad

7. Toss the chicken, noodles, cabbage, carrots, herbs and green onions

8. Toss with dressing and serve

Nutrition per serving: calories 373, 37g carb, 18g protein, 16 g fat, potassium 292 mg, phosphorus 154 mg, sodium 484 mg

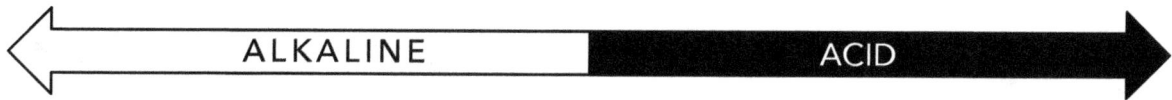

Strawberry Chicken Salad with Feta

SERVES 2

Ingredients

4	tsp olive oil (1 T plus 1 tsp) (you will use this divided in the recipe)
1	T white balsamic vinegar
1	tsp honey
½	tsp thyme
	Black pepper to taste
1	cups rinsed sliced strawberries
2	(3oz) skinless chicken breasts
½	tsp paprika
	Cooking spray
2	cups romaine lettuce
2	cups iceberg lettuce- see note regarding potassium at the bottom
¼	cup thinly sliced red onion
1	oz feta cheese

Directions

1. Combine 1 T oil, vinegar, honey, thyme, pepper and dash of salt in a medium bowl, whisk. Add ½ cup strawberries tossing to coat. Let stand for 10 minutes.

2. Heat a medium skillet over medium-high heat. Brush chicken with remaining tsp of oil, sprinkle with pepper and paprika. Coat pan with cooking spray, add chicken and cook 2-3 minutes on each side, or until done. Remove the chicken from the pan, let stand 5 minutes. Cut into slices.

3. Divide the romaine and iceberg lettuce, ½ cup strawberries and onion between 2 plates. Top with chicken and strawberry balsamic mixture.

4. Garnish with feta.

Nutrition per serving: calories 300, carbohydrates 12g, protein 29g, fat 16g, potassium 502 mg, phosphorus 283mg, sodium 432mg,

This recipe works better with baby spinach, **if your potassium is below 5.1** make it with baby spinach leaves instead of iceberg lettuce. **If potassium above 5.1: use iceberg lettuce.**

Green Bean Tuna Salad with Artichoke Hearts

SERVES 4

Ingredients

2   cups green beans

1   can light tuna packed in water- drained

½   purple onion chopped

4   marinated artichoke hearts chopped

2   T fresh dill

3   T lemon juice

3   T olive oil

1   garlic clove minced

1   tsp Dijon mustard

Directions

1. Place the red onion in ice water – this makes the flavor milder

2. Bring a pot of water to boil. Add the green beans and blanch for about 1-2 minutes or until bright green and just beginning to become tender. Pour into a colander and run cold water over them to stop further cooking.

3. Put the green beans in a bowl and add tuna, red onion, artichoke hearts

4. To make the dressing: in a bowl combine lemon juice, olive oil, garlic, dill, Dijon mustard, whisk well to combine

5. Pour the dressing over the salad and toss.

Nutrition per serving: calories 176, carbohydrates 12g, fat 11g, potassium 330 mg, phosphorus 115 mg, sodium 132 mg

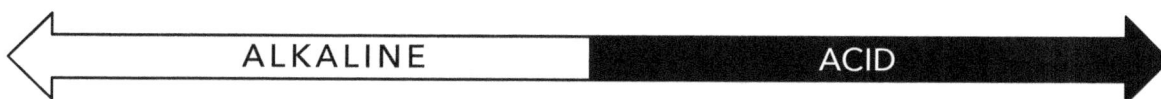

Greek Shrimp and Barley Salad

SERVES 8

Ingredients

Salad

1	lb shrimp, peeled and deveined
2	tsp olive oil
3	garlic cloves minced
3	cups low sodium chicken broth (make your own or buy commercial organic, additive free)
1	cup uncooked barley
2	cups cucumbers peeled and thinly sliced
1	cup grape tomatoes halved
½	cup cubed yellow bell pepper
⅓	cup feta cheese
¼	cup olives

Dressing

3	T olive oil
1	tsp grated lemon rind
2	T lemon juice
1	T minced fresh basil
1	tps fresh thyme minced
1	tsp red wine vinegar
½	tsp salt
3	garlic cloves, minced

Directions

1. Heat oil in a large skilled

2. Add garlic cook 1 minute till fragrant

ALKALINE   ACID

3. Add shrimp, sauté about 5 minutes till pink and done – set aside

4. Bring 3 cups broth to a boil in a large saucepan, add barley. Cover, reduce heat, simmer 35 minutes or until liquid has evaporated. Fluff with a fork and set aside to cool.

5. To make the dressing: combine oil, lemon rind, and remaining ingredients stir well.

6. Combine shrimp and barley, cucumber, tomatoes, bell pepper and olives and feta.

7. Add dressing to barley mixture, toss. Cover and chill.

Nutrition per 1 cup serving: calories 230, protein 18g, carbohydrates 18g, fat 3g, potassium 410 mg, phosphorus 249 mg, sodium 367mg

Blueberry Faro Salad

MAKES 4 HEARTY SERVINGS

If you have not tried faro, you will enjoy really enjoy it. The texture is a cross between rice and barley. Its good by itself or in a salad. This is a great combination of flavors and powerful antioxidants.

Ingredients

1	cup uncooked faro
2¼	cup vegetable broth- make your own or purchase an organic, additive free, lower sodium broth such as Pacific
2	large cucumber peeled and diced
2	cups fresh blueberries
2	T fresh mint chopped
⅓	feta cheese crumbled
¼	cup pistachios chopped
⅓	olive oil
¼	cup lemon juice

Directions

1. Rinse faro and place in a pan, add broth. Bring to a boil, reduce heat, cover and simmer for 25 minutes or until tender. Drain and set aside to cool.

2. Place the cooled faro into a bowl, add diced cucumber, blueberries, mint, feta cheese and pistachios.

3. Whisk together olive oil, lemon juice and pinch of salt and pepper

4. Toss the salad with dressing, let stand for 15-20 minutes and serve.

Nutrition per 1 serving: calories 421, carbohydrates 33g, protein 10g, fat 23g, potassium 316mg, phosphorus 230 mg, sodium 385mg

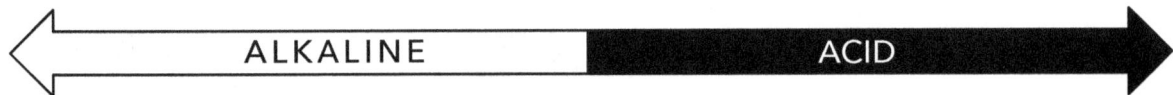

Taco Salad

SERVES 6

Ingredients

2	T olive oil
1	Onion- large chopped
1½	cups corn kernels
4	tomatoes chopped (use will be divided)
1½	cups brown rice – cooked
1	15 oz can black kidney beans- rinsed well
1	T chili powder (or more to taste)
1½	tsp dried oregano (divided)
½	cup fresh cilantro
⅓	cup prepared salsa
2	cups shredded iceberg lettuce
1	cup shredded jack cheese
2-3	cups coarsely crumbled tortilla chips

Directions

1. Cook brown rice according to package directions

2. Heat oil in pan. Add onion and corn cook for 5 minutes.

3. Add 1 of the chopped tomato, beans, cooked rice, chili powder, 1 tsp oregano to pan. Cook 5 minutes.

4. Coarsely chop the remaining 3 tomatoes, add cilantro ½ tsp oregano in medium bowl.

5. Toss lettuce in a large bowl, add bean mixture, half the fresh salsa 2/3 cup of the cheese. Serve sprinkled with tortilla chips and remaining cheese. Pass lime wedges and remaining salsa for extra garnish

Nutrition per serving: calories 311, carbohydrates 48g, protein 8g, fat 11g, potassium 489 mg, phosphorus 191 mg, sodium 281 mg

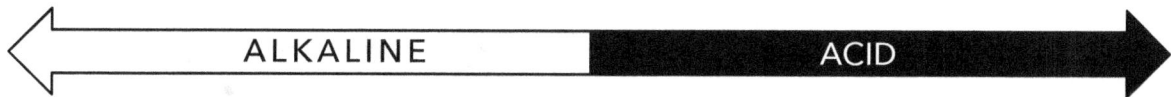

Mexican Style Quinoa Salad

SERVES 6

Ingredients

½   cup dry quinoa, rinsed

1   15 oz can black beans, drained and rinsed

1   cup salsa

8   oz corn- use frozen, allow to thaw

1   T chili powder

1   avocado peeled and diced

1   lime

Directions

1. Add 1 cup water to quinoa in a medium pot, bring to a boil. Reduce heat to a simmer, cover and cook until the moisture is absorbed, about 12-15 minutes. Turn off heat and let sit on stove for 5 minutes. Cool for 10 min or longer.

2. Add cooked quinoa, black beans, salsa, corn, avocado and chili powder. Toss to combine.

3. Squeeze the juice of 1-2 lime wedges over the salad, toss lightly

Nutrition per serving: calories 170, protein 8g, carbohydrates 28g, fat 4g, potassium 510g, phosphorus 177 mg sodium 410 mg.

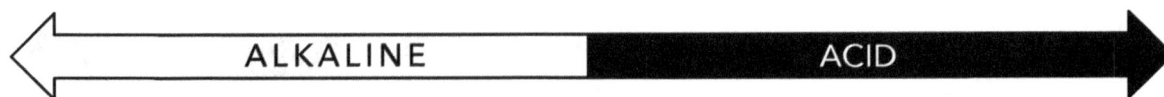

Greek Salad Layered Over Hummus and Pita

This can be a vegetarian meal or you can add chicken or shrimp- delicious,

SERVES 4 •1 PITA WITH HUMMUS AND SALAD

Ingredients

4	small whole wheat pitas
2	small tomatoes or 1 large cut into cubes
2	cups cucumber peeled and cubed
¼	cup crumbled feta
¼	red onion chopped
½	cup prepared hummus

Vinaigrette:

1	clove garlic
½	tsp dried oregano
¼	tsp Dijon mustard
2	tablespoons red wine vinegar
	Pepper to taste
4	tablespoons olive oil

Directions

1. To make the dressing: Place garlic, oregano, mustard, vinegar and pepper in a small bowl. Add olive oil in a slow stream and whisk as you are adding the oil.

2. Toast the pitas

3. Combine tomatoes, cucumber, feta, onion

4. Pour dressing over the vegetables- can let them sit for 30 minutes

5. Assemble: Place toasted pitas on plate, top with ¼ th of the hummus and ¼ th of the salad

Nutrition per serving: calories 233 cal, protein 5g, carbohydrates 18g, fat 3g, potassium 215 mg, phosphorus 107 mg, sodium 410 mg

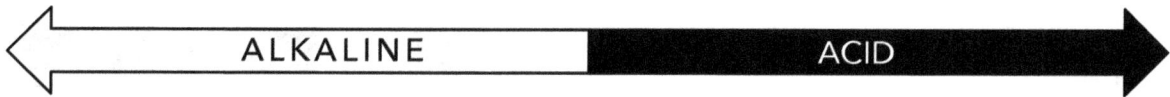

Lemony White Bean and Arugula Salad

SERVES 2

Ingredients

1   T olive oil

1   tsp grated lemon rind

2   T lemon juice

1   tsp Dijon mustard

     Black pepper to taste

1   cup cannellini beans, cooked

¼   cup thinly sliced red onion

2   cups raw arugula

Directions

1. Combine oil, grated lemon rind, lemon juice, mustard, and pepper in a large bowl, stirring with a whisk or fork.

2. Add beans and onions toss well to coat

3. Add arugula and serve

Nutrition per serving: calories 260, protein 10g, carbohydrates 26g, fat 14g, potassium 598 mg, phosphorus 126mg, sodium 247 mg

If your potassium is above 5.1: To reduce potassium substitute 1 cup of arugula for iceberg lettuce so the salad will be made from 1 cup arugula and 1 cup iceberg lettuce.

Lentil, Apple, and Walnut Salad
with Apple Cider Dressing

SERVES 8

Ingredients

1½	cup lentils
3	garlic cloves chopped
1	tsp dried thyme
1	bay leaf
2	cups apple cider
2	T Dijon mustard
2	T cider vinegar
2	shallots chopped fine
3	T canola oil
¼	tsp pepper
1	apple diced
8	cups baby spinach
½	cup chopped walnuts

Directions

1. Place in a large pot: lentils, garlic, thyme, and bay leaf cover with 2 inches of water. Bring to a boil then reduce to a simmer. Cook until tender but not mushy. Check after 15 minutes. Once done drain and rinse. Discard the bay leaf.

2. To make the dressing: in a sauté pan boil the cider until reduced to 1/3 cup. Allow the cider to cool.

3. Add the mustard, vinegar, shallots and oil, whisk until combined and emulsified

4. Season the dressing with pepper and pinch of salt. Toss the apples, lentils and spinach with the dressing garnish with walnuts, optional.

Nutrition per serving: calories 207, protein 11g, carbohydrates 31g, fat 5g, potassium 571, phosphorus 222mg, sodium 162mg

Guilt Free Guilt Free Ranch Dressing
with Assorted Vegetables

Ingredients

½   tsp dried onioins

½   tsp onion powder

½   tsp garlic powder

½   tsp salt

6   oz plain yogurt

Directions

1. Blend all ingredients together, stirring with a fork until throughtly mixed.

2. Add more onion or garlic as needed.

3. Serve with assorted vegetables of your choice

Nutrtion information per 1 oz: calories 20, carbohydrates 2g, fat 1g, potassium 76 mg, phosphorus 46 mg, sodium 189 mg.

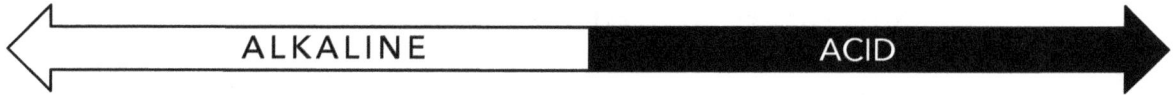

CHAPTER 14

Plant Based Main Course

Mexican Street Corn Tostadas

Black Bean Tacos

Roasted Eggplant with Tomatoes and Mint

Stuffed Portobello Mushrooms

Portabella Mushroom Burger

General Tso's Tofu

Egg Plant Teriyaki Stir Fry with Tofu

Lime Couscous with Assorted Vegetables

Black Bean and Butternut Squash Enchiladas

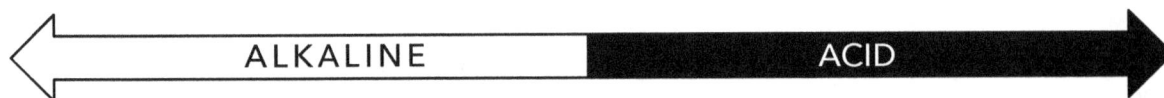

Mexican Street Corn Tostadas

SERVES 4 – 2 TORTILLAS EACH

Ingredients

8	(6 inch) corn tortillas	¼	tsp cumin
1	15 oz can black beans, rinsed and drained	2	T canola oil
¾	cups canned diced tomatoes with green chilies		
4	cups fresh or frozen corn kernels		
2	T sour cream	2	T mayonnaise
1	garlic clove minced	¼	tsp chili powder
2	T lime juice	½	cup feta cheese

Garnish: cilantro, green onion

Directions

1. Pre-heat oven 375. Line baking sheet with foil, arrange the tortillas in a single layer on the baking sheet. Mist with a vegetable oil cooking spray on both sides. Bake, flipping half way until they are crispy. Set aside (they will crisp more as they cool)

2. Combine black beans, diced tomatoes, cumin in a blender and blend but leave chunks.   (I like to use an immersion blender and blend directly in the pot- prior to heating)

3. Transfer beans to a pot and cook on medium heat for 15 minutes- set aside

4. Place the corn in a pan and heat

5. **To make the sauce:** combine sour cream, mayonnaise, chili powder, lime juice. Pour the sauce over the corn

6. **To assemble:** spread each tostada with ¼ of the bean mixture, top with ¼ of the corn mixture. Garnish with feta, cilantro and green onion

Nutrition info per 2 tortillas: calories 465, carbohydrates 66g, protein 16g, fat 18g, potassium 498 mg, phosphorus 304mg, sodium 401 mg

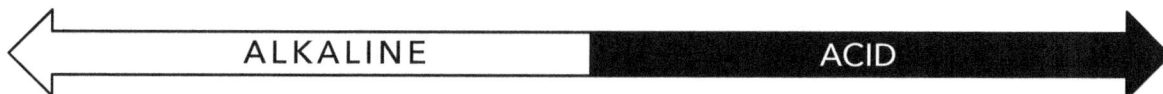

Black Bean Tacos

SERVES 4, 2 TACOS PER SERVING

Ingredients

8   flour tortillas

1½   cup cooked brown rice

1   lime

½   cup cilantro leaves

1   15 oz can black beans, rinsed and drained

2   cups arugula

1   cup salsa

Directions

1. Cook brown rice according to package directions.

2. Mix cilantro, lime juice and brown rice

3. Cook black beans in large pan until warm, add salsa stir and cook for 1 more minute

4. To make the taco use 1/8 of the rice mixture, 1/8 of the bean mixture, garnish with arugula and additional salsa

5. Garnish options: sour cream, cilantro, salsa

Nutrition information for 1 taco: calories 260, protein 10g, carbohydrates 46g, fat 4g, potassium 530mg, phosphorus 222 mg, sodium 489 mg

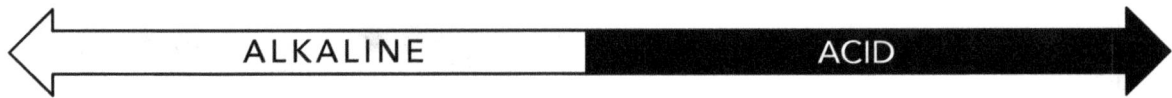

Roasted Eggplant with Tomatoes and Mint

This is a favorite dish of volunteer tasters- aka family and friends

SERVES 4

Ingredients

1-2   T + 4 tsp olive oil

1-2   lb eggplant (2 medium) cut into 1 inch slices

2   oz crumbled feta cheese

2   T capers

⅓   cup finely diced red onions

3   tomatoes- diced (1 ½ cup)

4   T mint leaves chopped

2   tsp red wine vinegar

       Black pepper to taste

Directions

1. Pre-heat oven to 425

2. Either spray each eggplant round with olive oil on each side or brush a large cookie sheet with olive oil.

3. Place eggplant on a single layer. Sprinkle with minimal salt and pepper.

4. Roast without disturbing 15-20 minutes. Flip and roast for another 10-15 minutes until soft and dark.

5. Mix feta, tomato, capers, onions, tomatoes, mint, vinegar and remaining 4 tsp olive oil in a small bowl.

6. Once the eggplant is done, top with tomato feta mixture.

7. Can be served as is or over whole wheat pasta or brown rice.

Nutrition per serving: calories 226, protein 5g, carbohydrate 17g, fat 15g, potassium 538 mg, phosphorus 114 mg, sodium 255 mg

Stuffed Portobello Mushrooms

2 SERVINGS : 2 MUSHROOM CAPS PER SERVING

Ingredients

4   Portobello mushrooms

3   T Balsamic vinegar

2   T olive oil

4   garlic cloves- chopped

½   onion- chopped

2   yellow pepper- chopped

2   tomatoes chopped

2   cups fresh spinach

¼-½ cup bread crumbs

2   T mixture of fresh oregano, basil, chopped

4   Mozzarella cheese slices

Directions

1. Pre-heat oven 375F

2. Remove stem and grill from mushrooms, use spoon to scoop it out

3. Brush the mushrooms with balsamic vinegar

4. Heat olive oil in small sauté pan. Add the onions and garlic, cook till translucent, add peppers, and cook till tender

5. Add tomatoes and spinach. Cook until spinach has wilted

6. Divide the filling and stuff the mushrooms

7. Sprinkle bread crumbs and Italian seasoning on top. Top with cheese

8. Place on a baking sheet and bake for 5-7 minutes or until the cheese has melted.

Nutrition per serving: calories 180, carbohydrates 8g, protein 6g, fat 8g, potassium 440mg, phosphorus 360 mg, sodium 120 mg

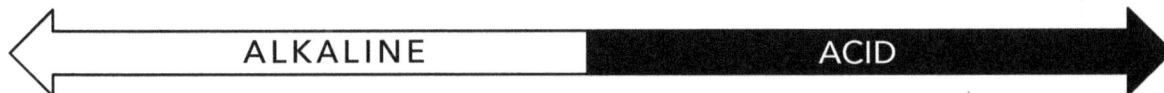

Portobella Mushroom Burger

SERVES 4

Ingredients

4   Portobello mushroom caps

2   T balsamic vinegar

1   T low sodium soy sauce

1   T olive oil

4   thick slices red onion

4   oz cheese swiss cheese

4   slices tomato

4   whole wheat hamburger buns

Directions

1.   In a large bowl whisk together vinegar, soy sauce, olive oil.

2.   Toss the mushroom caps with the sauce. Let stand at room temperature for 20-30 minutes

3.   Heat outdoor grill or pre-heat oven. Brush the grate with oil place the mushrooms on the grill or indoor oven and grill 7 minutes on each side or until done. Brush with marinade during cooking a few times.

4.   Grill the onion slices next to the mushrooms

5.   Place cheese on top of the mushrooms last 2 minutes.

6.   Assemble the buns, top with mushroom cap, onion and tomato

Nutrition: Serving size 1 loaded cap on bun: calories 295, carbohydrates 31g, protein 21g, fat 11g, potassium 441 mg, phosphorus 318 mg, sodium 493 mg.

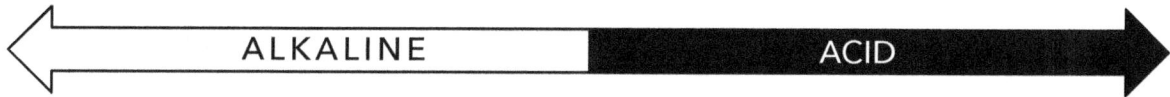

General Tso's Tofu

SERVES 4

Ingredients for the tofu

1	block extra firm tofu		4	T corn starch
2	T canola oil			

Sauce:

⅓	cup brown sugar		3	T hoisin sauce
3	T rice vinegar		2	T ketchup
2	T low sodium soy sauce		½	cup water
	Red pepper flakes to taste			

Garnish

1	T sesame oil		4	green onions
3	T fresh ginger grated			

Directions

1. Drain the tofu by wrapping a paper towel around it and putting a heavy object over it. Let it sit 20 minutes

2. In a bowl mix brown sugar, hoisin sauce, rice vinegar, ketchup and water red pepper flakes, set aside

3. Toss the tofu with the corn starch

4. Heat a skillet on medium heat, add 2T oil,

5. Place the tofu in the frying pan, cook until brown and crispy, remove from pan

6. Add sesame oil, onions and ginger. Cook until fragrant, add the sauce bring to a boil, simmer for 2 minutes. Add the tofu back to the pan and toss.

Nutrition per serving: calories 214, carbohydrates 7g, protein 11g, fat 15g, potassium 175mg, phosphorus 153 mg, sodium 466mg

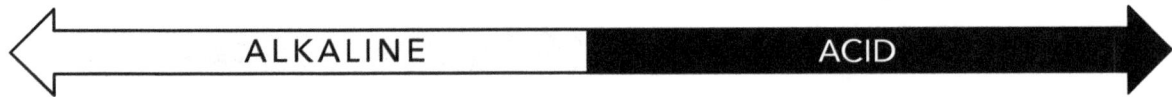

Eggplant Teriyaki Stir Fry with Tofu

SERVES 4

Teriyaki Sauce: Ingredients

⅓   cup balsamic vinegar

¼   cup maple syrup

1   T low sodium soy sauce

2   Tsp ginger- fresh, grated

1   garlic clove- crushed

1   tsp rice wine vinegar

⅓   cup water

Stir fry Ingredients

2   tsp canola oil

1   16 oz package tofu well drained, press to squeeze out excessive moisture, cut into cubes

1   lb Japanese eggplant (long and skinny) sliced into 1 inch cubes

¼   cup green onions chopped

1   garlic clove chopped

Garnish: green onions, sesame seeds

Directions

1. Combine the teriyaki sauce ingredient in a sauce pan and bring to a boil. Reduce heat and simmer for 15 minutes.

2. While sauce is cooking, heat 1 tsp oil in a large nonstick pan. Add the tofu and stir fry until golden for 5 minutes. Remove from the pan.

3. Add 1 tsp oil to pan, add eggplant, green onions, garlic and cook 5-10 minutes until soft. Add the tofu back in, add the teriyaki sauce and cook for 4-5 minutes.

4. Garnish with green onions and sesame seeds. Serve with ½ cup basmati rice or rice of your choice

Nutrition per serving with ½ cup rice: calories 324, protein 14g, carbohydrates 54g, fat 8g, potassium 460 mg, phosphorus 189 mg, sodium 162mg

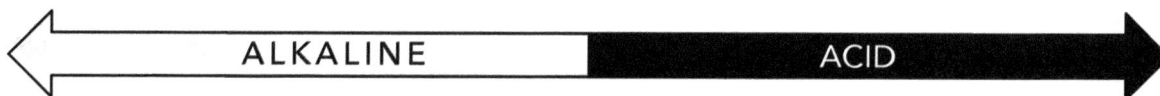

Lime Couscous with Assorted Vegetables

You can use be creative and use other vegetables of your choice or what is in season.

SERVES 6

Ingredients

10   oz package of couscous

3   cup home made or low salt organic chicken broth

1   T olive oil

2   cups coarsely chopped carrots

2   medium zucchini or yellow squash cut into ½ inch pieces

6   green onions cut into 1 inch pieces

Dressing

½   cup lime juice   ¼   cup olive oil

1   T honey   Pepper

½   cup chopped walnuts, toasted

2   oz parmesan cheese shaved or coarsely shredded

Directions

1.   Prepare couscous according to package directions or follow these directions:

2.   Bring 3 cups water or low sodium chicken stock, olive oil and dash of salt to a boil. Add the package of cous cous, or 1 ¼ cup. Turn off the heat and allow the cous cous to steam for 5 minutes. Let it rest until needed.

3.   In skillet add olive oil and heat, add carrots, cook 2 minutes.

4.   Add zucchini and green onions, cook 6 minutes.

5.   Transfer couscous to a bowl and add carrot, zucchini mixture.

6.   In a jar with a lid combine lime juice, olive oil, honey, pepper. Cover and shake well. Pour over the couscous, toss to combine. Garnish with walnuts and cheese

Nutrition information per serving: calories 383, carbohydrates 47g, protein 9g, fat 18g, potassium 499mg, phosphorus, 124 mg, sodium 45 mg

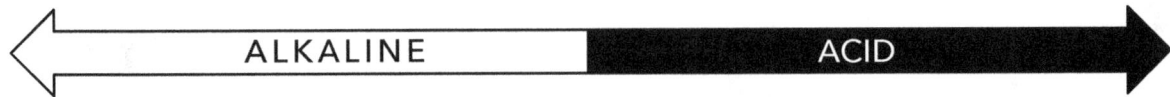

Black Bean and Butternut Squash Enchiladas

SERVES 8 • 2 ENCHILADAS EACH

Ingredients

1	cup uncooked rice- cook according to package directions
1	cup prepared red enchilada sauce
1	tsp olive oil
1	onion diced
3	cloves garlic minced
1	jalapeno seeded and diced
2	cups butternut squash- it can be found peeled and cubed in most grocery stores
1	10 oz can of chopped tomatoes with green chilis
¾	cups canned black beans
¼	cup water
¼	cup cilantro
1	tsp cumin
½	tsp chili powder
16	medium whole wheat tortillas
1	cup reduced fat shredded Mexican cheese
	Garnish: green onions, sour cream

Directions

1. Pre-heat oven to 400

2. Cook rice according to package directions

3. Heat olive oil in a large skillet, add onions, garlic and jalapeno. Cook 2 minutes.

4. Add the cubed squash, chopped tomatoes, black beans, water, cilantro, cumin and chili powder. Cook over low to medium heat, stirring every several minutes until squash in tender. About 30 minutes.

5. Add cooked rice to the mixture and combine well.

6. In a glass baking dish, place ¼ cup of enchilada sauce on the bottom and spread well

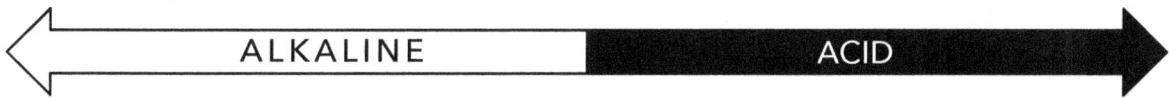

7. Place ⅓ cup filling in the center of each tortilla and roll

8. Place the tortilla in the glass baking dish, seam side down. Repeat with the rest of the filling and tortillas

9. Top with remaining enchilada sauce and cheese. Bake covered with foil for 10 minutes.

10. Garnish with scallions and sour cream and serve

Nutrition information per serving: calories 460, protein 14g, carbohydrates 80g, fat 9g, potassium 598 mg, phosphorus 301 mg, sodium 589 mg

This is a generous serving so 1 enchilada and a garden salad is fine for smaller appetites or if your potassium is above 5.1, have 1 enchilada and have a side of iceberg lettuce salad.

CHAPTER 15

Main Entree

Fish Tacos

Broiled Tilapia with Thai Coconut Curry Sauce

Salmon Bowl

Orange Maple Salmon

Dijon Salmon with Green Bean Pilaf

Baked Spaghetti Squash with Roasted Shrimp in a Lemon Sauce

Pesto Cauliflower Rice with Shrimp

Loaded Potato Skins with Black Beans and Ground Turkey

Turmeric Braised Chicken with Cauliflower and Leeks

Moo Shu Chicken Wrap

Fried Cauliflower Rice with Chicken

Fish Tacos

SERVES 4

Ingredients

8   oz white fish filet

1   T olive oil, divided

½   tsp chili powder

¼   tsp garlic powder

¼   tsp onion powder

4   corn tortillas

4   cups shredded cabbage (short cut use shredded cabbage for cole slaw in bag)

    Garnish: Pico de gallo or salsa, avocado chunks, cilantro,

Directions

1. Brush some oil on the fish, sprinkle with chili powder, garlic powder and onion powder on both sides.

2. Add olive oil to skillet and heat.

3. Add fish to the skillet cook 3 minutes per side or until the fish flakes easily with a fork.

4. Microwave the tortilla a few seconds till warm.

5. Place tortilla on plate add cabbage, pico de gallo, avocado, slices, top with fish, cilantro and serve.

Nutrition per 1 serving: calories 157, protein 13g, carbohydrates 16g, fat 5g, potassium 351mg, phosphorus 182 mg, sodium 50 mg

If your potassium is above 5.1 limit the avocado to 1 tablespoon or 1/8 of an avocado.

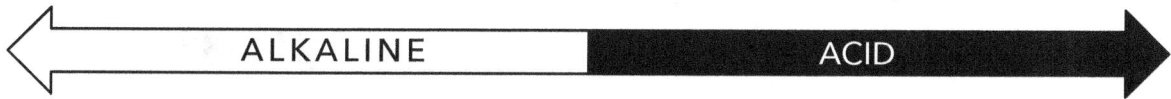

Broiled Tilapia With Thai Coconut Curry Sauce

SERVES 4 • 1 FILET, WITH ½ C SAUCE

Ingredients

1	tsp sesame oil, divided	2	tsp minced peeled fresh ginger
2	garlic cloves minced	1	cup red chopped red pepper
1	cup chopped green onions	1	tsp curry powder
2	tsp red curry paste (now found in most supermarkets)	4	tsp low sodium soy sauce
1	tsp ground cumin	1	T brown sugar
14	oz can light coconut milk	2	T fresh cilantro chopped
4	(6 oz) tilapia filets		Cooking spray
	Lime wedges		

Directions

1. Pre-heat broiler

2. In a large non-tick pan, heat ½ tsp sesame oil, add ginger and garlic. Cook 1 minute, add peppers and onions. Cook 1 minute

3. Stir in curry powder, curry paste, cumin. Cook 1 minute

4. Add soy sauce, brown sugar and coconut milk. Bring to a simmer (do not boil). Remove from heat, add cilantro

5. Brush fish with sesame oil, place fish on baking sheet coated with cooking spray. Broil 7 minutes or until is flakes easily.

6. Serve with lime wedge over basmati rice or rice of your choice.

Nutrition per serving of 1 filet with ½ cup sauce: calories 202, protein 32g, fat 6g, carbohydrates 6g, potassium 538 mg, phosphorus 258 mg, sodium 200mg,

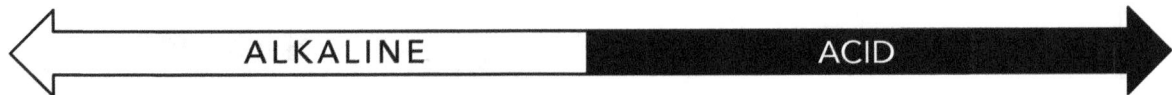

Salmon Bowl

SERVES 4

Fish and avocado are high in potassium. To reduce the potassium to 338 mg, omit the avocado. See note at the end of the recipe

Ingredients

½ cup green onions sliced

1 T sesame seeds

2 cups cooked brown rice

Olive oil spray

2 cucumbers peeled and chopped

1 avocado diced- see potassium note

16 oz salmon divided into 4 filets

For the vinaigrette:

2 T low sodium soy sauce

2 T mirin wine

1 T sesame oil

2 tsp wasabi in tube

2 T wine vinegar

Directions

1. Cook rice according to package directions- keep warm

2. Combine the vinaigrette ingredients in a bowl and set aside.

3. Season salmon with a pinch of salt and fresh pepper. Heat a frying pan or sauté pan over medium-high heat. Spray the pan lightly with oil spray. When hot sear salmon, around 2 – 4 minutes per side (depending on the thickness of the fish).

4. Split rice into four bowls equally, 1/2 cup each.

5. Top each bowl with 1 oz avocado, green onions, cucumbers, sesame seeds,

6. Place salmon on top of each bowl, drizzle with the vinaigrette

7. Serve immediately.

Nutrition per serving: calories 378, protein 19g, carbohydrates 22g, fat 21g protein 19g, potassium 707 mg, phosphorus 315 mg, sodium 330 mg

If your potassium is over 5.1: omit the avocado

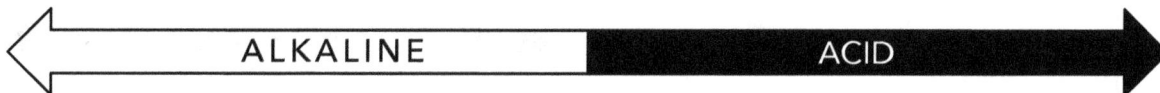

Orange Maple Salmon

SERVES 5

Ingredients

    Cooking spray

1.5   lb salmon fillets

1   T orange juice

2   T maple syrup

2   T Dijon Mustard- grainy type

2   tsp minced garlic

Directions

1. Pre-heat oven to 375

2. Spray baking pan with cooking spray and lay salmon fillet in dish, skin side down.

3. In a mixing bowl, whisk orange juice, maple syrup, mustard and garlic. Pour over salmon and cover with foil.

4. Bake for 15 minutes, uncover and bake another 5 minutes or until the top of the fish looks caramelized.

Nutrition Information Per serving: calories 210, protein 25g, carbohydrate 7 gm, fat 4 gm, potassium 450 mg, phosphorus 290 mg, sodium 180 mg

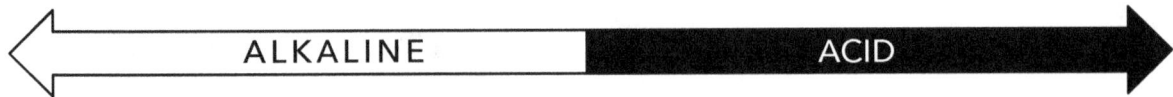

Dijon Salmon with Green Bean Pilaf

SERVES 4

Ingredients

1¼   lb salmon, skinned and cut into 4 portions

1   T minced garlic

2   T mayonnaise

½   tsp ground pepper divided

3   T olive oil- divided

    Pinch salt

2   tsp whole-grain Dijon mustard

Green Bean Pilaf

12   oz trimmed green beans

1   small lemon cut into 4 wedges, zest as well

7   oz brown rice, cooked

    Garnish fresh parsley

1   tsp crushed garlic

1   T pine nuts

2   T water

Directions

1. Cook brown rice according to pkg directions.

2. Pre-heat oven 425, line a baking sheet with foil or parchment paper

3. Brush salmon with 1T oil and place on baking sheet.

4. Mash garlic and salt into a paste with side of a knife, combine with mayonnaise, mustard and ¼ tsp black pepper. Spread the mixture on top of the fish

5. Roast the salmon until it flakes easily with a fork for 6-8 minutes per inch of thickness

6. Meanwhile heat the remaining olive oil in a large skillet, add the green beans, lemon, garlic zest, pine nuts. Cook until the green beans are tender. Reduce heat, add the cooked rice, water and cook 2-3 minutes or until hot.

7. Serve salmon garnished with parsley, accompanied by green bean pilaf

Nutrition per serving: calories 372, protein 31g, carbohydrates 17g, fat 21g, potassium 555mg, phosphorus 383mg, sodium 541mg

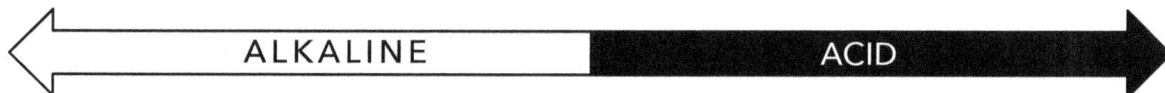

Baked Spaghetti Squash with Roasted Shrimp in a Lemon Sauce

SERVES 4

Ingredients

1	large spaghetti squash or 2 small			
12	oz shrimp peeled and deveined (20 shrimp)			
1	T olive oil	2	T butter
3	cloves garlic minced	1	tsp lemon zest
1	lemon juiced	1	tsp Dijon mustard
¼	tsp red pepper flakes	½	cup white wine
¼	cup half and half	2	T fresh parsley chopped

Directions

1. Cut spaghetti squash in half, place in microwave cook for 15 minutes

2. When cooked cut it open and let it cool so you can handle it.

3. Once cool scrape the strands and seeds from top of the squash till you reach the flesh. Scoop out the flesh into a bowl it will come out looking like spaghetti strands

4. In a large skillet, melt oil and butter over medium high heat, add shrimp and season with pepper, sautéing for 2 minutes. Add garlic and sauté for additional 1 minute until shrimp is cooked. Remove shrimp from the pan.

5. Add lemon juice and lemon zest, white wine, Dijon mustard and red pepper. Reduce heat and allow sauce to simmer for 5 minutes.

6. Cool sauce for 1 minute, add half and half and stir.

7. Assemble plates: If spaghetti squash too cool microwave to bring to desired temperature.

8. Place ¼ of squash on a plate, top with 1/4ᵗof the sauce and ¼ of the shrimp.

Nutrition information per serving: calories 168, protein 8g, carbohydrates 10g, fat 11g, potassium 219g, phosphorus 69 mg, sodium 138 mg

111

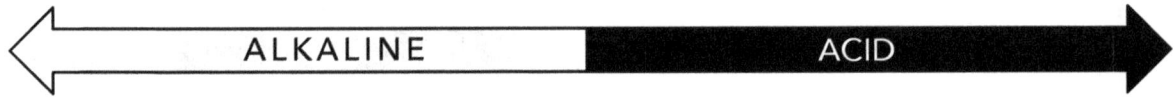

Pesto Cauliflower Rice with Shrimp

SERVES 2

Ingredients

1	tsp olive oil
½	lb peeled, devained shrimp
¾	cup cherry tomatoes cut into halves
12	oz cauliflower rice (found fresh or frozen at Trader Joe's, Whole Foods or regular grocery stores – frozen aisle by Bird's Eye)- no need to thaw or pre cook
¼	cup ready made pesto (check labels sodium content varies)

Directions

1. Heat a large frying pan over medium heat.

2. Once hot add olive oil and shrimp

3. Cook for 2-4 minutes until the shrimp start to turn pink on both sides- remove shrimp

4. Add tomatoes to the pan and cook for 1 minute

5. Add cauliflower frozen rice, cook until heated through, about 3-4 minutes. You want the cauliflower cooked but still crunchy.

6. Return shrimp to pan, add pesto sauce. With a spoon crush the tomatoes.

7. Remove from heat, can garnish with additional pesto or grated parmesan cheese.

Nutritional information per serving: calories 371, protein 34g, carbohydrates 10g, fat 22g, potassium 577mg, phosphorus 490 mg, sodium 510mg (may vary depending on sodium in ready made pesto sauce)

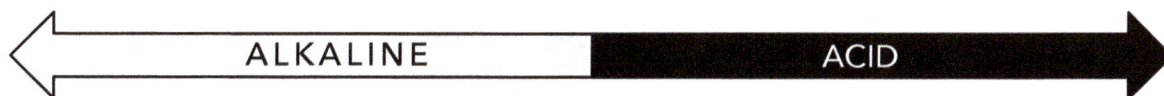

Loaded Potato Skins with
Black Beans and Ground Turkey

SERVES 4

Ingredients

2	medium baking potatoes	½	lb ground turkey meat
¼	chopped yellow onion	1	T garlic minced
½	cup black beans rinsed	½	cup corn
1	diced tomato		Cilantro
	Cumin		Cheddar cheese ½ cup shredded
	Sour cream		Pico de gallo

Directions

1. Bake potatoes in 350 F oven for 50 minutes or microwave for 10 minutes (pierce with fork prior to placing in microwave)

2. When potatoes are done cut in half, scoop out some of the inside to make room for filling but leave enough for yummy taste.

3. In a large skillet brown the turkey meat add onions, garlic, black beans, corn, diced tomatoes and cumin. Mix well and simmer covered for 20 minutes.

4. Add meat filling to potatoes top with shredded cheese. Place in oven till cheese has melted.

5. Serve with sour cream and pico de gallo

Nutrition: Serving half a potato with filling: calories 303, protein 23g, carbohydrates 29g, fat 11g, potassium 855 mg, phosphorus 357 mg, sodium 462 mg.

If your potassium is above 5.1 and you wish to reduce potassium in this recipe

Use either ground turkey or the black beans not both. Increase corn to make up the difference.

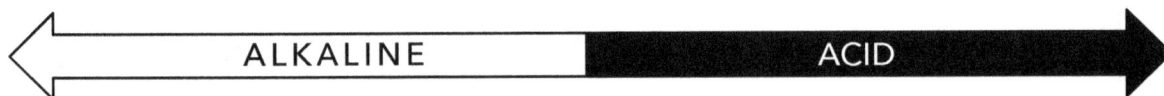

Turmeric Braised Chicken with Cauliflower and Leeks

SERVES 4

Ingredients

2	leeks
1	head of cauliflower cut into individual flowerets
2	tsp turmeric – divided
2	garlic cloves minced
1	tsp ground ginger
¼	cup fresh lemon juice
2	T olive oil –divided
4	skinless chicken drumsticks- on the bone
4	skinless chicken thighs on the bone
½	cup white wine (can also use chicken broth)

Directions

1. Preheat oven to 425 F

2. Slice the leeks in half-length wise, rise then well, fanning out the outer layers to get the sand and dirt. Slice the cleaned leaks into thin slices.

3. Chop the cauliflower into 1-2" flowerets

4. In a large mixing bowl toss the leeks, cauliflower with the garlic, 1 tsp turmeric, ginger, lemon juice and olive oil until combined. Save any unused marinade.

5. Spoon the mixture into a 9 X13 baking dish or casserole pan. Arrange in an even layer.

6. Add the chicken and the other tsp of turmeric to the mixing bowl and toss to coat in the remaining turmeric mixture.

7. Add to the casserole dish and nestle in the vegetable mixture. Drizzle with any remaining marinade.

8. Roast uncovered until the chicken is tender about 1 hour.

Nutrition per serving: Serving size is 1 drumstick and 1 thigh with 1/4th of the vegetable mixture: calories 272, fat 14g, protein 27g, potassium 486 mg, phosphorus 257mg, sodium 318 mg,

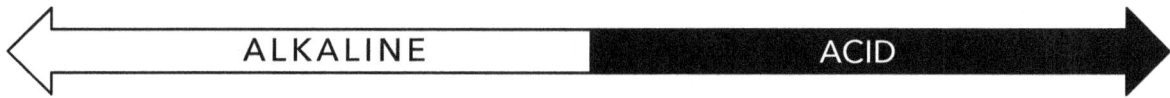

Moo Shu Chicken Wrap

SERVES 4

Ingredients

1	T dark sesame oil
1	T minced ginger
5	garlic cloves minced
1	cup carrots cut into matchstick size pieces
1	cup brown button mushrooms sliced
1	cup green onion cut into 1 inch pieces
4	cups prepared shredded cabbage (I buy coleslaw mix)
1	lb chicken breast thinly sliced
	Cooking spray
1½	T water
1	T hoisin sauce
8	(6.5 inch whole-wheat tortillas)

Directions

1. Heat a large skillet over medium heat. Add oil, swirl around to coat, add garlic and ginger cook 30 seconds.

2. Add carrots and mushrooms, cook 2 minutes, add onions and cabbage, cook 2 minutes or until cabbage wilts- remove to a large bowl

3. Coat pan with cooking spray, add chicken cook 2-3 minutes on each side until browned and done.

4. Add water to pan and scrape pan to loosen browned bits. Add hoisin sauce.

5. Add cabbage back to pan toss to combine.

6. To make the roll up: Add 2/3 c of chicken-cabbage mixture on top of each tortilla, roll up and enjoy.

Nutrition per serving of 2 tortillas: calories 473, protein 26g, carbohydrates 65g, fat 13g, potassium 580 mg, phosphorus 267mg, sodium 426mg,

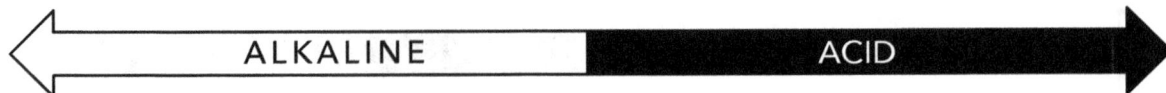

Cauliflower Fried Rice

SERVES 4

Cauliflower rice is all the rage and available fresh or frozen in many grocery stores. I prefer the frozen and have found it at Trader Joe's, Whole Foods as well as my local chain grocery store. Bird's Eye makes it and can be found in freezer section with other frozen vegetables.

Ingredients

1	tsp peanut oil and 2 T divided
2	eggs beaten
3	scallions sliced
1	T fresh ginger grated
1	T garlic minced
1	lb boneless chicken breast or thighs cut into 1 inch pieces
½	cup diced red pepper
1	cup snow peas
4	cups frozen cauliflower rice
3	T soy sauce reduced sodium
1	tsp sesame oil

Directions

1.   Heat 1 tsp oil in a large skillet. Add the beaten eggs and cook without stirring until fully cooked on one side. Flip and cook 30 seconds on the other side and remove from heat. Cut into inch pieces

2.   Add 1 T oil to pan along with scallions, ginger and garlic. Cook for 30 seconds, add chicken and cook for 1 minute, add bell pepper, snow peas, stirring until just tender about 1-2 minutes. Remove from heat

3.   Add remaining 1 T oil to pan, add the cauliflower rice and heat on high heat until soft but crunchy

4.   Return chicken mixture and eggs to pan, add soy sauce and sesame oil. Stir till well blended. Garnish with more scallions.

Nutrition per 1 serving: calories 304, carbohydrates 12g, protein 30g, fat 15g, potassium 575 mg, phosphorus 241 mg, sodium 401 mg. The major contributor of potassium in this recipe is the chicken.

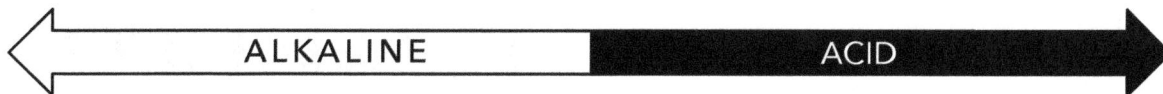

Sheet Pan Chicken Fajitas

SERVES 5 • 2 FAJITAS EACH

For the marinade:

2	tablespoons lime juice		2	tablespoons fresh cilantro
½	red onion chopped		¾	tsp dried oregano
½	cup vegetable oil		1	lb chicken breasts cut into strips

Spices for vegetables

1	tsp chili powder		½	tsp cumin
½	tsp garlic powder		1	T olive oil
1	large red bell pepper sliced		1	large yellow pepper sliced
2	cups sliced onions		10	corn tortillas warmed

garnish lime wedges, cilantro, sour cream

Directions

1. The day before is best but at least few hours before serving. In a large zip lock bag combine lime juice, cilantro, onion, oregano and vegetable oil, add the sliced chicken. Refrigerate overnight.

2. One hour before toss vegetables with chili powder, cumin, garlic powder and oil let sit

3. Pre-heat oven to 400

4. Arrange the chicken and vegetables on a sheet pan, bake for 15 minutes

5. Turn oven to broil and broil until the chicken is cooked and vegetables are slightly browned in spots – 5-7 minutes

6. Squeeze lime juice over chicken and vegetables

7. Serve the chicken and vegetables with warmed tortillas garnished with cilantro, lime wedges and sour cream

Nutrition per 2 fajitas served on 2 corn tortillas: calories 329, protein 34g, carbohydrates 31g, fat 8g, potassium 540, phosphorus 379, sodium 514 mg

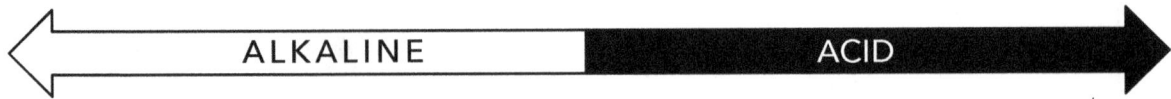

Cuban Chicken with Coleslaw

SERVES 4

Ingredients

4	small chicken breasts, boneless or bone in your choice
¼	cup lemon juice
2	tablespoons lime juice
2	tablespoons fresh cilantro
½	red onion chopped
2	tsp orange zest (orange peel cut into tiny pieces)
¾	tsp dried oregano
¾	cup vegetable oil
5	cloves garlic minced

Directions

1. Combine all ingredients, add chicken. Pour marinate, add chicken in large zip lock plastic bag or glass pan, cover and refrigerate at least 2 hours or overnight.

2. This recipe is best on grilled outside 7 minutes each side for boneless and up to 11 minutes on each side for bone in. Test a small piece of chicken to make sure no pink remains.

3. You can also bake it in a 375 oven for 30 minutes. Test to make sure it is cooked thoroughly.

Nutrition information per serving: calories 201, protein 24g, carbohydrate 2g, fat 3g, potassium 306mg, phosphorus 191mg, sodium 60 mg

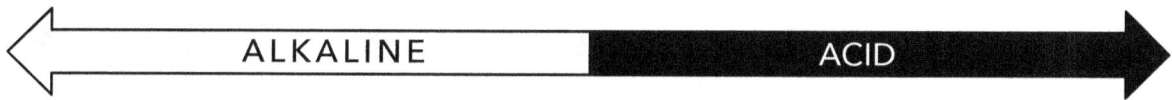

Southwestern Coleslaw

SERVES 10 • SERVING SIZE 1 CUP

Ingredients

7   cups shredded green cabbage (can buy short cut shredded cabbage)

3   carrots, peeled and grated

1   red pepper seeded, cored, diced

3   scallions chopped

1   small jalapeno seeds discarded, chopped fine

Dressing

¼   cup apple cider vinegar

1   T lime juice

1   T honey

2   tsp chipotle salt free seasoning

⅓   cup olive oil

½   cup toasted pecan pieces

Directions

1.   In a large bowl combine the cabbage, carrots, red pepper, scallions and jalapeno. Toss well

2.   In a small bowl, whisk together vinegar, lime juice, honey, and chipotle seasoning. Add the olive oil in a slow stream while whisking to emulsify. Pour the dressing over cabbage mixture and mix well.

3.   Garnish with pecans and serve

Nutrition per 1 cup serving: calories 140, carbohydrates 10g, protein 2g, fat 11g, potassium 265 mg, phosphorus 50 mg, sodium 35 mg

ALKALINE   ACID

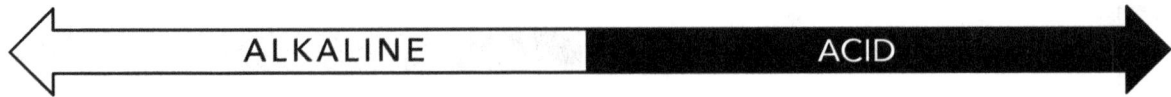

Korean Grilled Chicken

SERVES 4

The flavor of this marinade is soo good and its so easy.

Ingredients

1   lb (2 boneless chicken breasts) cut in half

⅓   cup low sodium soy sauce

¼   cup unsweetened applesauce

¼   cup yellow onion chopped

1   tsp sesame oil

1   tsp grated ginger

1   T brown sugar

2   garlic cloves crushed

1   tsp red pepper flakes

1   tsp sesame seeds

2   scallions chopped

Directions

1. Place the chicken in a ziploc plastic bag and pound to an even thickness, about ½ inch

2. In a bowl, combine soy sauce, applesauce, onion, sesame oil, ginger, brown sugar, garlic, red pepper flakes, sesame seeds. Reserve ¼ cup marinade. Transfer the rest of the marinade into a plastic Ziploc bag, add the chicken. Refrigerate for at least 4 hour or overnight.

3. Heat the grill, spray with nonstick grill spray. Place the chicken on the grill. Cook for 4 minutes and turn the chicken, top with more marinade. Cook additional 4 minutes or until done.

Nutrition per serving: calories 180, carbohydrates 9g, protein 25g, fat 4g, potassium 160 mg, phosphorus 94mg, sodium 495 mg

120

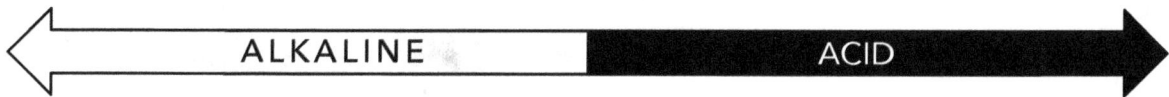

Moroccan Marinated Chicken

SERVES 8

Ingredients

4	Tbsp olive oil
4	Tbsp lemon juice
3	cloves garlic
1	tsp coriander
¼	tsp cumin
1	tsp paprika
⅛	tsp chili powder
	Pepper to taste
½	bunch parsley
½	bunch cilantro
4	skinless chicken breasts

Directions

1. Put all ingredients in zip lock bag, add chicken and refrigerate overnight.

2. Grill approximately 7 minutes per side, test small piece to make sure done. Or Bake at 375, covered in oven, uncover and cook additional 15 minutes.

Nutrition per serving: calories 180, carbohydrates, 1g, protein 25g, fat 4g, potassium 158 mg, phosphorus 94 mg, sodium 195 mg

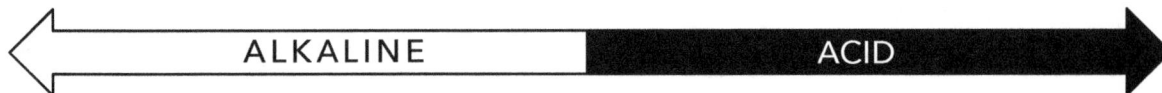

Scrumptious Marinade

SERVES 6

Ingredients

6	small/medium chicken breasts
¼	cup cider vinegar
3	tablespoon Dijon mustard
3	garlic cloves
¼	cup lime juice
½	cup lemon juice
½	cup brown sugar
6	tablespoons olive oil

Directions

1. Place all ingredients in zip lock bag, add chicken and refrigerate overnight.

2. Grill approximately 7 minutes per side, test a small part to make sure its done

3. Or bake at 375, covered in oven, uncover and cook additional 15 minutes.

Nutrition per serving: calories 178, carbohydrates 4g, protein 25g, fat 4g, potassium 158 mg, phosphorus 88 mg, sodium 182 mg

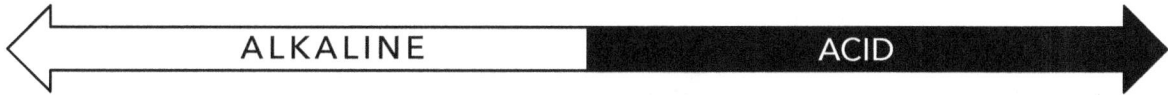

ALKALINE   ACID

CHAPTER 16

Dessert

Chocolate Cherry Bars

Plum Cake

Peach Tart

Stove Top Summer Fruit Crisp

Baked Apples

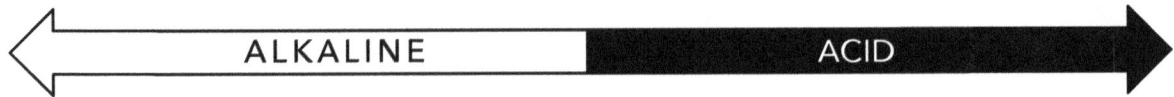

Chocolate Cherry Bars

Diabetic appropriate

SERVES 16

Ingredients

2½ cup unsweetened puffed wheat cereal	½ cup pecan halves, chopped
⅓ cup roasted pepitas (pumpkin seeds)	¼ cup dried cherries or cranberries
2 T sesame seeds	1 T flax ground flax seeds
½ cup honey	½ tsp vanilla extract
⅛ tsp salt	½ cup semisweet chocolate chips

Directions

1. Position the rack in lower third of the oven, preheat 300F.

2. Line cookie sheet with parchment paper

3. Toss cereal with pecans, pepitas (pumpkin seeds), cherries or cranberries, sesame seeds and ground flaxseeds in a large bowl,

4. In a small sauce pan, combine honey, vanilla and salt. Warm over medium heat until the honey is more fluid. Pour the honey over the dry ingredients and fold until all combined.

5. Let cool for 5 minutes and fold in chocolate chips.

6. Scrape the mixture onto the cookie sheet with parchment paper. Spread evenly with a fork. If too sticky you can cover with another piece of parchment paper and use that to press into the cookie pan.

7. Bake for approximately 35 minutes (or less to make sure the honey does not burn)

8. Cool for 1 hour in the refrigerator

9. Using the parchment paper, lift off the pan, peel the paper and cut into bars or squares.

Nutrition per 1 serving: 109 calories, 5 g fat, 17 g carbohydrates, 1 g protein, 66 mg potassium, 45 g phosphorus, 110 mg sodium

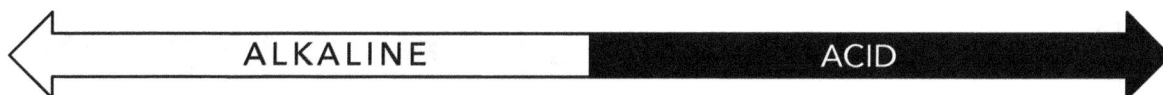

Plum Cake

SERVES 10

This cake is easy and you can use different flavor mixes; butter, pineapple, coconut, vanilla. Try different fruit including apricots, peaches, nectarines or berries . Add orange or lemon zest. This cake is moist and the fruit adds a nice sweetness so you don't need to top with frosting which decreases total fat and sugar.

Ingredients

1   box cake mix (yellow, vanilla, pineapple or coconut)

       purple plums halved and pitted

Directions

1. Preheat oven to 350, using a glass square 8-inch pan spray with cooking nonstick spray

2. Prepare cake according to directions

3. Spread half the cake mix in the pan, top with all the plums, squishing them together to make room for all.

4. Top with the remaining cake batter

5. Bake 40 minutes- test with a toothpick (insert into center of cake if comes out clean your cake is done. If comes out with some cake stuck to it bake another 5-6 minutes and test again)

Nutrition per serving: calories 238, protein 4g, fat 4g, carbohydrate 49g, potassium 128 mg, phosphorus 200 mg, sodium 446mg

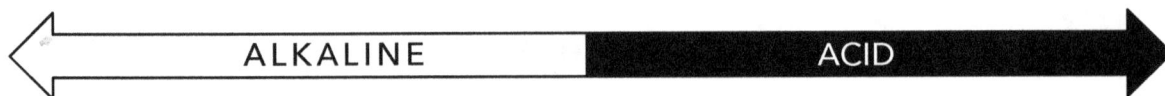

Peach Tart

SERVES 6

Ingredients

½	refrigerated unbaked piecrust
¼	cup sugar
4	tsp flour
¼	tsp ground nutmeg
3	cups sliced peaches (1 ½ lb)
1	T lemon juice
1	egg beaten
1	tsp water

Directions

1. Pre-heat oven 375

2. Let the piecrust stand at room temperature- according to package directions.

3. Line a cookie sheet with foil and sprinkle lightly with flour

4. Unfold the pastry sheet and place on the foil

5. In a large mixing bowl, stir sugar, flour and nutmeg. Stir in the peaches and lemon juice.

6. Spoon the peach mixture on top of the crust. Leave a 2-inch border. Fold the pastry border over the peaches (just the edges)

7. Beat the egg and 1 tsp water, brush the tart with the egg mixture

8. Bake 40 minutes until golden. If you see the pastry browning too quickly, top with tin foil the last 10 minutes.

Nutrition per serving: calories 112, carbohydrates 24g, protein 2g, fat 2g, potassium 245mg, phosphorus 31 mg, sodium 123 mg

Stove Top Summer Fruit Crisp

SERVES 6

Ingredients

2	tsp unsalted butter
1	lb strawberries sliced
1½	cup raspberries (divided)
1½	cup blackberries (divided)
1	T brown sugar
½	tsp vanilla extract
¾	cup low fat granola
	Optional yogurt, frozen yogurt

Directions

1. Melt butter in a large skillet over medium heat

2. Add strawberries, 3/4 cup raspberries, ¾ cup blackberries, sugar, vanilla to pan.

3. Cook 4 minutes or until fruit starts to soften. Stir in remaining berries, cook 1 more minute.

4. Divide berry mixture between 6 bowls. Top with granola.

5. Optional: Add frozen yogurt or regular yogurt

Nutrition per serving (no yogurt): calories 131, carbohydrates 29g, protein 3g, fat 2g, potassium 315mg, phosphorus 77mg, sodium 37mg

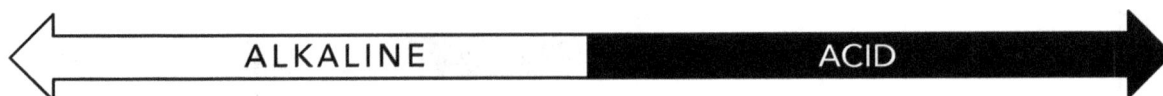

Baked Apples

SERVES 4

Ingredients

2   large apples – I like Granny Smith

2   T butter melted

2   T brown sugar (if you want to reduce sugar use Brown Sugar Splenda)

2   T flour

4   T quick cooking oats

     Dash of cinnamon

Directions

1. Pre-heat oven to 375

2. Cut apples in half and remove the core

3. In a bowl combine butter, brown sugar flour, oats and cinnamon

4. Spoon on top of the apple halves and sprinkle with cinnamon

5. Place the apples of a cookie sheet and bake for 30 minutes

6. Serving size in ½ apple

Nutrition per serving: calories 153, protein 1g, carbohydrates 26g, fat 6g, potassium 168 mg, phosphorus 42mg, sodium 5 mg

ALKALINE ← → ACID

Recipe Index

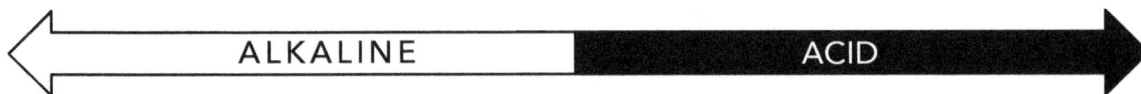

Dessert

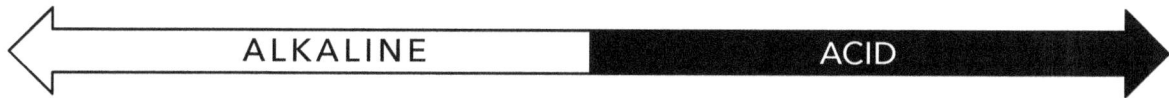

ALKALINE ACID

References

Caravaca F1, Villa J, García de Vinuesa E, Martínez del Viejo C, Martínez Gallardo R, Macías R, Ferreira F, Cerezo I, Hernández-Gallego R. *Relationship between serum phosphorus and the progression of advanced chronic kidney disease Nefrologia.* 2011;31(6):707-15. doi: 10.3265/Nefrologia.pre2011.Sep.11089.

Hess, Bernhard. (2006). *Acid–base metabolism: implications for kidney stone formation.* Urological research. 34. 134-8. 10.1007/s00240-005-0026-0.

Anna Gluba-Brzozka, Beata Branczyk and Jacke Rysz *Vegetarian Diet in Chronic Kidney Disease- A Friend or Foe.* Nutrients 2017 Apr 9 (4): 374. Published online 2-17 Apr 10. Doi.

Philippe Chauveau MD, Christian Combe MD, Denis FougueMD, Michel Aparicio MD. *Vegetarianism: Advantages and drawbacks in Patients with Chronic Kidney Disease.* Journal of Renal Nutrition, Vol 23, no 6 (November), 2013: pp 399-405

Nimrit Goraya,[*†] Jan Simoni,[‡] Chan-Hee Jo,[*§] and Donald E. Wesson[⊠*†] *A Comparison of Treating Metabolic Acidosis in CKD Stage 4 Hypertensive Kidney Disease with Fruits and Vegetables or Sodium Bicarbonate.* Clin J Am Soc Nephrol. 2013 Mar 7; 8(3): 371–381.

Kamyar Kalantar-Zadeh, Lisa Gutekunst, Rajnish Mehrotra, Csaba P.Kovesdy, Rachelle Bross ,Christian S. Shinaberger, Nazanin Noori, Raimund Hirschberg,Debbie Benner, Allen R. Nissenson†, Joel D. Kopple *Understanding Sources of Dietary Phosphorus in the Treatment of Patients with Chronic Kidney Disease.* Clinical Journal of the American Society of Nephrology. March 2010 vol 5 no3 519-530.

Ivana Lazich MD, George L.BakrisMD *"Prediction and Management of HyperkalemiaAcross the Spectrum of Chronic Kidney Disease"* Seminars in Nephrology Volume 34, Issue 3, May 2014, Pages 333-339

Sharon M. Moe, Mirian P. Zidehsarai, Mary A. Chamgers, Lisa A. Jackman, J. Soctt Radcliffe, Laurie L. Trevino, Susan E. Donahue, John R. Asplin. *Vegetarian Compared with Meat Dietary Protein and Phosphorus Homeostasis in Chronic Kidney Disease.* Clinical Journal of the American Society of Nephrology. February 2011 vol 6 no 2 257-264

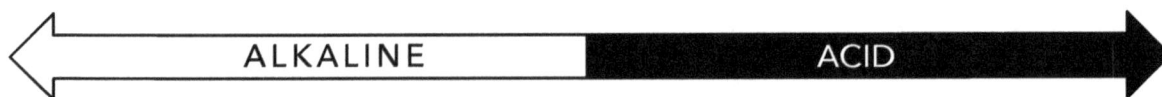

Musso CG: Potassium metabolism in patients with chronic kidney disease (CKD): Part I—Patients not on dialysis (stages 3–4). Int Urol Nephrol 36: 465– 468, 2004

Remer T, Manz F. Paleolithic diet, sweet potato eaters, and potential renal acid load. Am J Clin Nutr. 2003;78(4):802–803

Remer T, Manz F. Estimation of the renal net acid excretion by adults consuming diets containing variable amounts of protein. Am J Clin Nutr. 1994;59(6):1356–1361

Raphael KL, Wei G, Baird BC, Greene T, Beddhu S. Higher serum bicarbonate levels within the normal range are associated with better survival and renal outcomes in African Americans. Kidney Int. 2010;79(3):356–362

Phisitkul S, Hacker C, Simoni J, Tran RM, Wesson DE. Dietary protein causes a decline in the glomerular filtration rate of the remnant kidney mediated by metabolic acidosis and endothelin receptors. Kidney Int. 2008;73(2):192–199

Schwarz S, Trivedi BK, Kalantar-Zadeh K, Kovesdy CP: Association of disorders in mineral metabolism with progression of chronic kidney disease. Clin J Am Soc Nephrol 1: 825– 831, 2006

Scialla JJ, Appel LJ, Astor BC, et al. Net endogenous acid production is associated with a faster decline in GFR in African Americans. Kidney Int. 2012;82(1):106–112

Scialla JJ, Appel LJ, Wolf M, et al. *Plant Protein Intake is Associated With Fibroblast Growth Factor 23 and Serum Bicarbonate Levels in Patients With Chronic Kidney Disease: The Chronic Renal Insufficiency Cohort Study*. J Ren Nutr. 2012;22(4):379–388. e371

Shubha K.De' XiaoboLi, Manoj Monga, Department of Urology, Glickman Urological and Kidney Institute, Cleveland Clinic, Cleveland, *Changing Trends in the American Diet and the Rising Prevalance of Kidney Stones. Urology* Volume 84, Issue 5, November 2014 pages 1030-1033

Sullivan CM, Leon JB, Machekano R, et al. Effect of food additives on hyperphosphatemia among patients with end-stage renal disease. JAMA 301 : 629-635, 2009

Jaime Uribarri and Man S, Oh The key to halting progression of CKD might be in the produce market, not the Pharmacy. Kidney International (2012) 81. 7-9

Wesson DE, Jo C-H, Simoni J. Angiotensin II receptors mediate increased distal nephron acidification caused by acid retention. Kidney Int. 2012 Epub ahead of print.

Wesson DE, Simoni J, Broglio K, Sheather S. Acid retention accompanies reduced GFR in humans and increases plasma levels of endothelin and aldosterone. Am J Physiol Renal Physiol. 2011;300(4):F830–837.

Potassium in Food Additives: Something Else to Consider; Editorial, Journal of Renal Nutrition Vol 19, no 6 (November), 2009; 441-442

National Institutes of Health, National Center For Complementary and Integrative Health. Soy Information

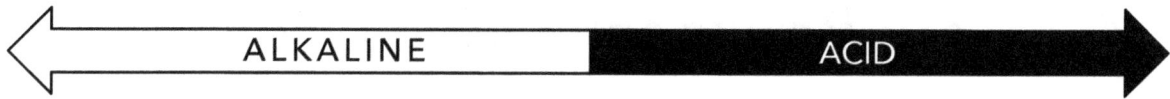

About the Author

Nina Kolbe RD CSR LD has been a practicing dietitian for over 22 years. She has chosen to specialize in kidney disease and became one of the first dietitians in the country to take the board certification exam to earn the title of Certified Renal Specialist. To maintain this certification 75 hours of continuing education must be maintained in the field of kidney disease. This assures the patients that they are receiving the most up to date information from their health professional.

Nina Kolbe maintains a private practice with many physicians in the Washington DC metro area referring to her for nutritional counseling. In addition to a private practice Nina also serves on the medical steering committee board of National Institutes of Health Kidney Disease Education Program, the medical steering committee of the National Kidney Foundation. She has been the chairperson for Council of Renal Nutrition, a Renal Dietitian group for 3 years.

Nina Kolbe has conducted research in the field of renal nutrition. She has presented her research at the National Kidney Foundation's Clinical Meetings. She has been published in the medical journal, Nephrology News & Issues. Nina frequently presents lectures to health professionals in the field on renal nutrition.

This passion and dedication to her profession stems from the belief that early diagnosis, medical and nutritional intervention can delay the progression of kidney disease and depending when treatment is started, avoid dialysis.

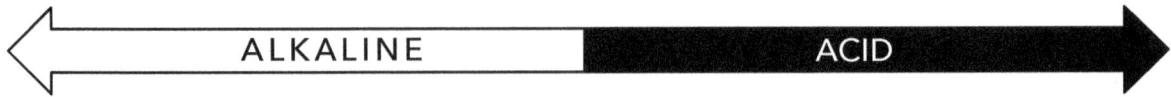

More Books for Kidney Health

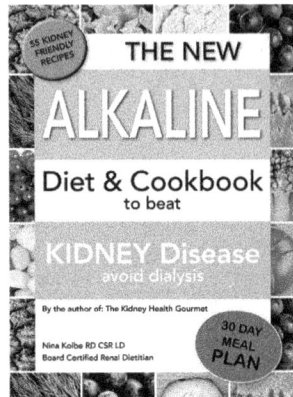

Improve kidney health with the new Alkaline Diet and Cookbook. 30 days meal plan, change the way you eat and take charge of your health

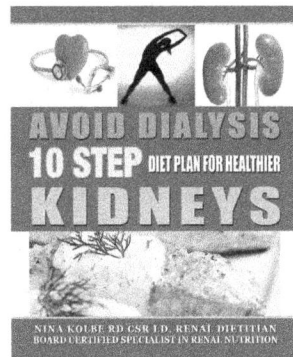

Take charge of your kidney disease, understand your laboratory values. Learn what your protein needs, potassium, sodium and phosphorus needs are. Sample meals, supplements and hot of the press research

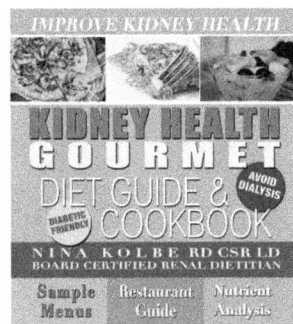

More than just a cookbook. A guide to selecting everything from beverages, snack, breakfast cereals and lettuce. Recipes adapted for chronic kidney disease with nutrient analysis

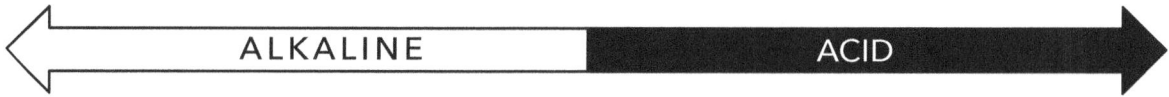

ALKALINE ACID

Order By **Mail:**

Nina Kolbe

215 E Street SE

Washington, DC 20003

Phone: 202-390-8044

Email: ninakolbe@icloud.com

www.kidneyhealthgourmet.com

I would like to order _____ copy of The New Alkaline Diet & Cookbook $12.99, $4.00 shipping

I would like to order _____ copy of Avoid Dialysis, 10 Step Plan. $12.99, $4.00 shipping $16.99

I would like to order _____copy of Kidney Health Gourmet $12.99, $ 4.00 shipping, $16.99

Save on shipping buy 2 or more and pay just $4.00 shipping for the entire order

Name   _____

Mailing Address   _____

_____

Telephone   _____

Email   _____